Curable Hypertension: Primary Aldosteronism

Janet Walberg Rankin, Ph.D.

DEDICATION

This book is dedicated to the many undiagnosed individuals who have primary aldosteronism. The stories of those who have gone years without diagnosis and appropriate treatment are heartbreaking, unnecessary, and inspired me to write this book. Personally, I dedicate this book to my husband and friends who helped me during my own period of turmoil when I was without a diagnosis.

TABLE OF CONTENTS

ACKNOWLEDGMENTS

I thank the many teachers throughout my education who helped instill my curiosity, love of learning, and doggedness to get to the bottom of a problem. I have also learned from my many students and particularly thank Michelle Smith Rockwell, R.D. who provided insightful suggestions for an early draft of this book. I appreciate the many scientists and clinicians who are studying primary aldosteronism and hope that their work expands and translates to improved understanding and treatment for this condition. Specifically, I would like to thank Dr. John W. Funder who replied to me with encouragement from far Australia when I wrote to him in appreciation for his bold impact on PA. The fact that Dr. Robert M. Carey was willing to take a look at the manuscript for accuracy and write a Foreword for this book astonishes and humbles me. His leadership in developing consensus for hypertension treatment guidelines is extraordinary. Dr. Clarence Grim impresses me as he unselfishly provides daily free advice to people searching for answers about PA. Amazingly, I have not met any of these physicians in person. Yet it is clear that they are dedicated scientists and physicians who have taken their commitment to heal patients to the highest level.

FOREWORD

Hypertension (high blood pressure), the world's leading risk factor for morbidity and mortality, is one of the most prevalent medical conditions. Hypertension affected one-quarter of the world's adult population – nearly one billion people - in the year 2000 and its prevalence is projected to rise to 29% by 2025. The current prevalence of hypertension in the United States is 28% but it is even higher (30-45%) in European countries. In the United States, hypertension is the most common reason for visiting a physician for ongoing medical care. The prevalence of hypertension is directly proportional to age; more than half of Americans over age 65 have high blood pressure. Strikingly, the remaining lifetime risk of developing hypertension for men and women who are not yet hypertensive by middle age is 90%.

High blood pressure is a major risk factor for cardiovascular disease (coronary artery disease, myocardial infarction and congestive heart failure), cerebrovascular disease (stroke) and end-stage kidney disease. Blood pressure is continuously related to these risks even down to a normal blood pressure of 115/75 mm Hg. That is, the higher the blood pressure, the higher the risk. For example, each increase of 20 mm Hg systolic blood pressure or 10 mm Hg diastolic blood pressure doubles the risk of a fatal cardiovascular event.

Suboptimal blood pressure control is the most common attributable risk for death worldwide, being responsible for 62% of strokes, 49% of coronary heart disease and over 7 million deaths per year. Indeed, hypertension ranks third in disability-adjusted life years worldwide. However, the risk of cardiovascular disease can be greatly reduced or even eliminated with effective antihypertensive therapy.

Lifestyle changes (weight control, reduction of salt intake, stopping alcohol consumption, etc.) are important adjuncts to treatment, but the vast majority of hypertensive patients require daily antihypertensive medications taken for a lifetime to control their blood pressure. Even then, only about half of treated hypertensive patients have their blood pressures adequately controlled according to 2008 statistics.

Unfortunately, the vast majority of hypertensive patients, over 90%, have primary (essential) hypertension resulting from a combination of genetic and lifestyle factors that cannot be specifically diagnosed or treated. Blood pressure can only be controlled with medications in these patients. However, about 10% of patients have secondary hypertension for which a definable cause can be found and, in many cases, the hypertension can be improved or even completely eliminated with specific treatment.

By far, the most common form of secondary hypertension is primary aldosteronism, currently estimated to be present in about 8-10% of all hypertensive patients and 20% of those with drug-resistant hypertension. The hypertension in these patients is due to over-production of the adrenal hormone aldosterone. In about one-half of these patients, high aldosterone secretion is from a small, benign tumor in the outer layer of the adrenal gland. For these patients, surgical removal of the adrenal gland improves and often cures both the hypertension and the detrimental organ damage caused by excessive aldosterone production. In the remaining 50%, treatment with a specific drug class [mineralocorticoid (aldosterone) receptor antagonists] can have a similar beneficial effect. The main barrier to finding patients with primary aldosteronism is knowing when and how to screen for this condition. Unfortunately the possibility of primary aldosteronism is frequently overlooked, for years or even decades, imposing a major health risk for these patients.

Clinical guidelines for physicians published by the Endocrine Society (*Journal of Clinical Endocrinology and Metabolism*) in 2008 and updated in 2015 provide authoritative physician education on the diagnosis and management of primary aldosteronism. However, patients with hypertension, especially those with uncontrolled or drug- resistant hypertension, also need to be aware of the possibility that their hypertension might be caused by primary aldosteronism. A question from such a patient on the appropriateness of screening for primary aldosteronism would be welcomed by most, if not all, primary care physicians.

Curable Hypertension: Primary Aldosteronism is a reliable resource for patients with hypertension and/or primary aldosteronism. It is a well-written, authoritative and timely volume intended to help hypertensive patients be cognizant of and understand primary aldosteronism. The book reviews the prevalence, pathogenesis, diagnosis, disease subtypes, medical and surgical treatment and ongoing care of primary aldosteronism from the patient's perspective. It provides valuable information about what patients should expect at each step along road to diagnosis and treatment.

This book is written by a patient for patients. Janet Walberg Rankin, however, is an unusually sophisticated patient in that she possesses an extensive scientific background and the ability to translate complex medical concepts and terms into clearly understandable information for the lay reader. Dr. Rankin is Professor of Human Nutrition, Foods and Exercise at Virginia Tech University in Blacksburg, Virginia. She received her PhD degree in Nutrition from the University of California Davis in 1982 when she joined the faculty at Virginia Tech. She has published over 50 articles on nutrition and sports medicine and was President of the American College of Sports Medicine in 2012. We are fortunate that Dr. Rankin has made a commitment to educating patients based on her own personal experience as a patient. I recommend this book as a valuable resource for patients with hypertension, for patients undergoing diagnostic evaluation for primary aldosteronism, to help with their decision making capacity, and for patients in whom primary aldosteronism requires a partnership with their physician in the process of disease management.

Robert M. Carey, MD, MACP
Professor of Medicine (Endocrinology and Metabolism)
Dean, Emeritus
University of Virginia School of Medicine
April 10, 2015

Chapter 1

WHAT'S THE PROBLEM?

"You are the healthiest person I know," said one of my friends, incredulous that I had been diagnosed with high blood pressure that would sometimes swing to over 200/100 mm. I was similarly perplexed but also anxious to understand why I was experiencing this problem.

Ultimately, I determined I had a serious medical condition that is estimated to affect up to eight million people with only about 1% of them getting appropriate treatment [27]. This seems outrageous based on our advanced medical establishment but the data backs this up. Could you be one of the 99% who have been plagued for years with symptoms such as headache, muscle cramps, blurry thinking, and blood pressure that is difficult to control even when you are taking multiple medications? It is possible that you have a condition—primary aldosteronism (PA)--that disproportionately increases your risk of heart attack, heart rhythm abnormalities and stroke. The good news is—there are highly effective treatments! We need to get these treatments to more people.

I wrote this book to provide a resource that I would have wanted when I was struggling with a set of unusual problems that were stumping my physicians. Even after the diagnosis, I could not find any books written for the public on this condition. I was lucky that I had an alternative way to find information about the condition. Working as a faculty member at a university and having enough training in the health sciences to understand most medical research papers, I eventually found my "cure." I am now passionate about helping to reach some of the 99% who could be released from scary, debilitating, and dangerous symptoms.

There are numerous posts on the Internet about the long delay in correct diagnosis and treatment. "It took 20 years to get a diagnosis". "In the 9 years prior to the PA diagnosis…". Some of the frustration in delayed diagnosis is expressed below:

> *My first PC [primary care] doctor was a "wait-and-see" doctor. Try a new pill, wait-and-see. Try another new pill, wait-and-see. Try these pills together, wait-and-see. We did that for 2 years. Once I switched doctors my new PC immediately tested for aldosterone and within 5 months of switching doctors I was cured. (Freeste)*

> *There are so, so many uneducated doctors out there and too many who are all too anxious to write us all (PA patients) off as being hypochondriacs…. Would you believe I had a scan done years before I was dx'd [diagnosed] but that particular endocrinologist dismissed the tumor as NOT being related to my high bp and low potassium so I went several more years with multiple trips to the ER and one hospitalization for the low potassium (1.8 - critically low), panic attacks & high blood pressure. (Susie)*

I observed Internet postings that describe undergoing many years of medical care without successful resolution of symptoms. A study of one clinic over a 30- year period, measured 7.6 years delay in primary care, with an additional 1.5 years delay in a hypertension clinic before correct diagnosis and management of patients with PA [18]. Another study reported that patients diagnosed with PA had hypertension for an average of 10.1 years before diagnosis [34]. When they received the appropriate treatment, many experienced what they described as a "miracle cure" and a "life-changing" experience. However, the longer people went without the correct treatment, the less likely they were to have substantial improvement in the negative consequences of the disease.

By educating physicians and the public, we should be able to reduce this unnecessary period between development of problematic symptoms and correct diagnosis. The right treatment is highly effective, can cure the problems experienced by most people, and can prevent some of the very serious medical side- effects of living with undiagnosed PA.

This book is not meant to substitute for good medical care with a physician. I am completely clear that I am not a physician and can only supplement information you might be getting from a licensed doctor. This book represents my understanding as an educated layperson and I cannot verify the complete accuracy of my interpretations. My philosophy is that it is best to be well informed and work with your medical team to determine the optimal path to health. I hope this book will help with that. This is not a physician-bashing book. My father was a physician; my brother is a physician. My point is that some doctors were trained years ago when PA was considered rare. Much of the information in this book has been discovered in the last 10-20 years. If your physician has stayed current in this area, that's wonderful. If not, you need to be more involved in your health care.

This book is organized to help you understand the prevalence and cause of this condition, describe who is likely to get it, how it is diagnosed, the best treatments, and tips for living with PA. I begin with my own story to provide my perspective and reason I tackled the writing of this book. It will use some terms that will be further defined and described in the latter sections (go to the glossary in this book for definitions for many terms). I have acquired the information in this book through countless hours of reading medical papers as well as the interaction with other people with this disease or those who treat it. I have purposely provided the scientific references for many of the statements so that those who are interested can read the original articles. The scientific and medical sources are provided in bracketed numbers throughout the text with the full list in the "References" section.

Quotes from the Internet are used in the book to provide examples of personal experiences. They are presented as posted with the exception that identifying information has been deleted. Only quotes that I was able to contact the individual and get their permission were included. I have altered their user names, if requested. I have not altered their words but sometimes provide a definition for an abbreviation in brackets.

It was crucial for me to understand the physiology and science of PA, but I understand that might not fascinate or be important to you. In general, I have used (but also defined) many of the appropriate technical, medical terms because this could help you better understand your physician and medical tests. I have provided a glossary as well as some tables defining terms or abbreviations that may be unfamiliar. In fact, some terms have been defined multiple times since I am sensitive to the fact that these may be unfamiliar to many readers. I have separated the most complicated information in "Technical Discussions" that you can ignore, if you choose, or come back to later. If you don't have much interest in understanding the scientific basis for this disease or diagnosis, you could jump right to the chapter, "Living with PA", for practical suggestions. Finally, since science is always evolving, I am using a portion of the proceeds to develop and maintain a website to provide updated information as medical science and treatment continues to evolve: https://primaryaldosteronism.wordpress.com/.

Chapter 2

MY STORY

As a 58 year- old female in 2013 with no personal risk factors or family history of heart disease, I expected to face cancer at some point, but development of a cardiovascular problem never entered my mind. To support that assumption, I have always had low-normal blood pressure, lipids, glucose, and body fat. I had healthy behaviors— I have never smoked, have always been highly physically active, have eaten in a healthy manner. As a university professor in a department of "Human Nutrition, Foods, and Exercise," it was almost considered part of the job to have healthy behavior.

Yet during a routine health screening required for new health insurance in September 2013, the technicians measured my blood pressure as 150/90 mm. Although that is not imminently dangerous, it was definitely highly unusual for me. I had a completely normal blood pressure reading (116/70 mm) just 15 months earlier at my doctor's office. In fact, I was smug enough to dismiss it as likely defective equipment and didn't think another thing about it until the following week when I had previously scheduled my annual gynecological exam. The office nurse noted the same high blood pressure. Now I was worried.

I assumed this "out of the blue" increase in BP was due to some secondary cause since I did not have the characteristics of someone with primary hypertension (*e.g.*, obesity, inactivity, family history). In addition, since I had not seen a progressive rise in blood pressure over time, this seemed to be related to some new problem. A visit to my primary care physician within a week confirmed the high blood pressure. My doctor encouraged me to start measuring and recording blood pressure using a home system I purchased at a local store.

He initially prescribed three drugs (losartan, HCTZ, carvedilol)--- and later increased the doses when there was no beneficial effect on my blood pressure. He also tried a fourth drug, amlodipine, but I went off this after a few days when I experienced a never-before felt, startling fluttering heart at night. No lifestyle changes were suggested except that I should not do any high intensity exercise until my blood pressure was more controlled.

In spite of the medications, my blood pressure was volatile and unpredictable. Sometimes it was normal, but many days it would rise to 150-180 mm. Sometimes I would wake in the middle of night with systolic pressures over 200 mm with symptoms of burning in my heart, jitteriness, feverishness, and a general sense that I was about to have a serious cardiac or stroke event. My doctor told me to take another beta-blocker pill (carvedilol) in these cases, but he didn't seem concerned. The drugs had a very modest effect on reducing these high pressures (about 10 mm). These episodes scared me and I was glad to have my husband there in case I had a more serious event.

Although the doctor believed this might be primary hypertension that had developed due to my age, I just could not believe this was the case because of my lack of risk factors or family history and apparent sudden onset. In order to search for any causes of secondary hypertension (blood pressure caused by another primary problem, see Chapter 3), he had me do a 24-hour urine collection, to test for vanillylmandielic acid (diagnoses pheochromocytoma, a tumor in adrenals producing too much epinephrine, see Chapter 3)—my value was is in the normal range so we eliminated this as a cause. My routine blood work was normal, so this excluded a thyroid problem (another cause of secondary hypertension).

My doctor suggested a renal artery duplex, an ultrasound test that evaluates the blood flow in kidney, to check for renal artery stenosis (narrowing of arteries leading to kidney, another cause of secondary hypertension). This test suggested some modest narrowing of the left renal artery. Although this test is known to be a rather rough estimate of kidney blood flow, we jumped on this as a possible answer to my problems. The next step in verifying whether this was the cause of my hypertension was to do a more invasive, expensive test. An angiogram involves injection of a dye into the renal arteries to view them after catheterization through an artery in the groin.

While waiting for this to be scheduled, my symptoms continued to get worse and more frequent. Along with the high blood pressure, I experienced muscle twitching and cramping, constipation, jitteriness and a feeling of feverishness, sleeping problems, and sporadic chest discomfort (tightness) that alerted me of an increase in my pressure. I avoided exercise—highly unusual for me—since I worried it would make things worse.

In late December, I was scheduled for a renal artery angiogram. The doctor would follow the angiogram with angioplasty—ballooning the artery open—if he found narrowing. As I was awake during the procedure, I heard the doctor say, "I don't see anything." Although he later said he did not see any stenosis (narrowing of the renal arteries) that would cause blood pressure trouble, he did angioplasty on one spot that he thought looked slightly narrowed, just in case.

I hoped this modest change would be a cure. Although my blood pressure was good for the two days I was in bed recovering after the angioplasty, it quickly went back to old pattern once I was up, about and eating and moving as usual. So I was back to "square one".

One comment the interventional radiologist had in his notes from the angiography procedure was that he could see I had some "excessive vasculature" between left adrenal and kidney that I should have further evaluated. I'm not sure what he suspected, but my primary care doctor ordered an abdominal computed tomography scan (CT) with contrast in early January to explore this. (See descriptions in Chapter 5 for more detail on what is involved with this test.) The radiologist reported no problems with the adrenals from the CT with the exception of minor pericardial effusion (extra fluid around the heart).

Now my doctor and I were discouraged. He suggested visiting a cardiologist to see if he had any insights. In the meantime, not ready to completely give up, I delved into the medical literature on resistant hypertension to see if there was something we were missing. My scientific training in physiology and health was very helpful in being able to understand most of the basics in these articles. I found multiple articles and studies that showed a benefit of a drug I had not tried, spironolactone, for "resistant hypertension."

I asked my doctor if I could try this medication that is often used for people with PA, a condition we had not tested for. I suggested he measure my ratio of blood aldosterone to renin (see later discussion in diagnosis section) since I had read enough to realize that this is recommended before beginning the medication. He approved trying the new drug (although he suggested using a similar drug, eplerenone, instead of spironolactone) but did not agree to the blood sample since he said it would not make any difference in my treatment. So later that day, I began 25 mg/d of eplerenone.

Within days, this drug had a quick and wonderful effect. I felt better in every way and my blood pressure started to improve. Within a week, my systolic pressures were 110-130 mm about every day, down from the typical 150-170 mm it had been. I could sleep through the night, did not feel the tightness/burning in my heart that accompanied swings in blood pressure, and was less jittery and feverish. What a relief! I had found the appropriate treatment and believed I had PA, although without the baseline blood sample, I did not have a definitive diagnosis.

I went ahead with the visit to the cardiologist that had already been scheduled. Similarly, he did not seem to know much about PA nor believe I likely had it. Because of the pericardial perfusion (excess fluid between the heart and the lining of the chest wall) noted in my abdominal CT, he asked for an echocardiogram. This test showed some dilation (expansion) of the atria (upper chambers of the heart), modestly reduced ejection fraction (proportion of the blood in the heart ejected with each beat), and the curious pericardial effusion previously seen in the CT scan. I was to see him in six months for a repeat echocardiogram.

I began reading everything I could find on PA to more fully understand this condition and to see if this was likely the cause of my problems. I also found several on-line chat groups that shared experiences and suggestions related to this condition. My initial symptoms and reaction to the eplerenone—the only drug that seemed to be effective—convinced me this is what I had. I came to believe the swings in blood pressure I experienced were due to changes in the sodium content of my diet. It seemed that the days I experienced severely high blood pressure were days I had eaten high sodium foods. Obviously, I am not a doctor and did not have the data (blood tests) to be confident that this hunch was correct. To have a true diagnosis, I now understood I would have to go off eplerenone for at least 4-6 weeks to go through a battery of tests (described later). Having finally found a "cure," I was not motivated to do this.

As long as I tolerate the drugs and maintain stability, I believe I will continue with the medical treatment that is working for me. One modification I made was to try dropping the beta-blocker, carvedilol. I dropped this over a week, cutting the dose each day, and had no change in my blood pressure. I had also increased my dose of eplerenone to 50 mg per day since I had a few episodes of high blood pressure, sometimes after I had exercised earlier in the day or maybe eaten more sodium than usual. This dose appears to be effective virtually every day for me while I maintain a reduced sodium diet.

In retrospect, I believe that PA should have been the first thing the doctor checked since, as you will read later, it is the most common cause of secondary hypertension. Overall, I feel lucky that it only took about five months after development of symptoms for me to get the appropriate treatment. Some patients undergo many, many years of inappropriate, ineffective treatments before they are diagnosed.

The idea for this book came about when I realized there was no easily accessible, comprehensive resource for patients with PA. I read all the summaries in medical Internet sites like WebMD but craved more information. I wanted to understand why I might have this, what my risks were, and how I could best live with it. I had many questions—if I had this, why was something not seen on the CT scan? How important was dietary sodium restriction? What were my risks of heart attack and stroke? Was it important for me to get a definitive, legitimate diagnosis of PA or could I simply continue with the medication regimen?

Scientific and medical journals had a wealth of information that helped me with these questions. Since these resources are either not available or difficult to interpret by the majority of individuals, I decided to create this book to summarize what I understand about the causes, tests, and treatments for PA and provide some guidance on living with this disease.

Chapter 3

THE SURPRISING PREVALENCE OF
HYPERTENSION AND PRIMARY ALDOSTERONISM

How Common is Hypertension?

Most of you know that the top cause of death in the US is cardiovascular disease (heart disease and stroke), accounting for about 32% of all deaths in 2010. Since there is not a single measurement that will determine who will get cardiovascular disease, we use a set of "risk factors" as predictors (Table 1). Some risk factors are considered "major" meaning they substantially increase risk. Hypertension (high blood pressure) is one of these. In fact, since it is so common (one out of every three adults and the majority of those over 55 years in the US have hypertension) and strongly increases risk, it is the top contributor in the US population, of all the risk factors, to development of cardiovascular disease.

Hypertension is a major public and personal health problem. The latest estimate is that 80 million people in the US, about one third of all adults, have hypertension [55] with about 17% unaware that they have it (Figure 1). The prevalence of hypertension goes up with age so that about 65% of adults over the age of 65 years have high blood pressure. Hypertension is more common in African Americans than other races. More men have hypertension than women before the age of 45 years, but more women have hypertension after the age of 64.

Table 1. Risk Factors for Cardiovascular Disease

Cannot Change	Changeable
Age	Smoking
Male gender	Hypertension
Heredity	Dyslipidemia (high blood cholesterol and low blood high-density lipoprotein, HDL)
	Inactivity
	Diabetes or pre-diabetes

Figure 1. Proportion of Hypertensive Individuals Who Know They Have High Blood Pressure

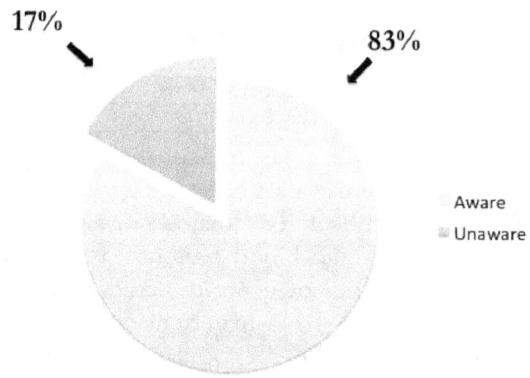

Have High Blood Pressure

17%

83%

Aware
Unaware

If high blood pressure is detected, your medical team will try to bring your blood pressure to normal levels to reduce your risk of stroke, kidney damage, and coronary heart disease. Unfortunately, many people (about 14 million) with hypertension are unaware that they have it. Only about half of those who know they have hypertension are in "control," meaning that their blood pressure is at acceptable levels. This leaves about 16 million people in the US who know they have high blood pressure but have not been able to reduce it to normal through treatment (Figure 2).

Figure 2. Status of Individuals Who Know They Have High Blood Pressure

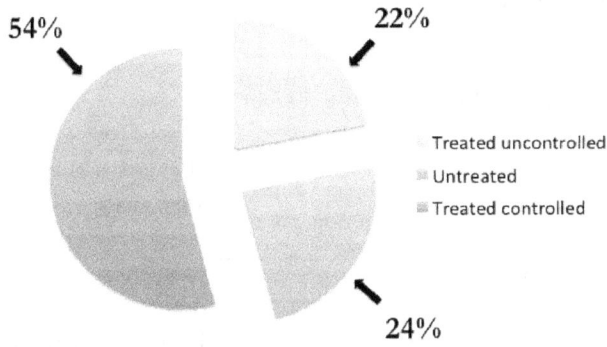

Treated? Controlled?

54%

22%

Treated uncontrolled

Untreated

Treated controlled

24%

Blood Pressure Targets—What is "Normal"?

Blood pressure is always given as two numbers. The first, higher number is the systolic blood pressure while the second is the diastolic blood pressure. The systolic is the higher pressure since this occurs when blood is pumped out of the heart into the blood vessel system. The diastolic blood pressure is the pressure in the vessels between heart contractions. The pressure is measured in millimeters (mm) of mercury (Hg, is the chemical symbol). Most people just quote the numbers, like 120 (systolic) over 90 (diastolic) when referring to blood pressure.

Doctors look to official recommendations regarding acceptable levels for blood pressure. The National Institutes of Health (NIH) has administered the National High Blood Pressure Education Program for over 30 years. This group, made up of professional and public organizations, along with federal agencies, appoints a committee (called the Joint National Committee, JNC) to discuss and produce recommendations on the targets for blood pressure based on the best available evidence. Physicians use these reports to determine which patients need treatment as well as the target blood pressures to be achieved through treatment.

Recommendations of a committee appointed to JNC-8 were published in 2014 [42], updating the recommendations of 2003 (JNC-7) [43]. Modifications in these new guidelines received a lot of attention and have been controversial. Regardless, the JNC-8 recommendations changed several recommended blood pressure goals and procedures, including the advocated blood pressure to be less than 150/90 mm for those 60 years and older and less than 140/90 mm for adults younger than 60 or those with diabetes or kidney disease. This compares to the previous JCN-7 goal of less than 140/90 mm for those older than 50 and less than 130/80 mm for adults younger than 50 and for those with diabetes or kidney disease (Table 2).

Table 2. Latest JCN-8 Blood Pressure Targets

Group	Target Blood Pressure
Younger than 60 years	Less than 140/90 mm
Older than 18 with diabetes or kidney disease	Less than140/90 mm
60 years or older	Less than150/90 mm

The opinion of the JCN-8 group was that previous lower targets were not supported by strong evidence and that too many patients with hypertension, especially older individuals, are over-treated in order to achieve a particular blood pressure goal. Drug treatment can have negative side effects that the committee felt were unacceptable. I will not debate the value of this change in blood pressure targets but share this so you are aware of the latest recommendations available to your physician. It also is of interest to point out that the NIH is no longer involved in developing any clinical guidelines as of June 2013, so this report was published independent of the federal agency.

You may hear the term "prehypertension" to refer to blood pressure that is greater than 120/80 mm but less than the cut off for hypertension. The American Heart Association also provides designations to describe the severity of hypertension (Table 3).

Table 3. American Heart Association Categories for Hypertension

Category	Systolic Pressure, (mm)		Diastolic Pressure, (mm)
Normal	Less than 120	and	Less than 80
Prehypertension	120-139	or	80-89
Stage 1 hypertension	140-159	or	90-99
Stage 2 hypertension	160 or higher	or	100 or higher
Hypertensive crisis	180 or higher	or	110 or higher

Most Common Causes and Treatment of Hypertension

Blood pressure is a measurement of the sideways pressure of the blood against the walls of the arteries—similar to the pressure of water released from a faucet on the sides of a hose. Blood pressure can be too high for two primary reasons:

- The small arteries, called arterioles, constrict so that their diameter is reduced.
- The volume of blood in the circulation is expanded, pushing harder against the vessel walls.
- Sometimes, both of these conditions are at play to increase blood pressure.

About 75% of individuals with diagnosed hypertension are taking medications. The most common types include: diuretics, angiotensin converting enzyme inhibitors (ACEi), angiotensin receptor blockers (ARB), beta-adrenergic blockers, and calcium channel blockers. Each of these types of medications works to reduce either blood volume or blood vessel constriction. (Medications are discussed in detail in Chapter 7.)

Lifestyle changes including diet, physical activity, and stress reduction are also recommended as part of the treatment for all hypertensive patients according to the American Heart Association and the American College of Cardiology [20].

What is Resistant Hypertension?

When you have tried three or more medications and still have not reached blood pressure goals, you can be classified as having resistant hypertension (Table 4). Some individuals with apparent resistant hypertension may actually not be complying with their medication prescriptions—forgetting or purposely not taking them regularly. Others who remain hypertensive in spite of three or more medications may be resistant because their form of hypertension isn't "fixed" by the medications they are taking. For example, they may have PA but have not received the appropriate treatment.

Table 4. Types of Hypertension

Primary Hypertension (also called "essential hypertension"): high blood pressure due to no defined cause but typically associated with obesity, poor diet, sedentary lifestyle, and family history

Secondary Hypertension: high blood pressure caused by another medical condition

Resistant Hypertension: blood pressure that does not achieve target levels in spite of three or more medications

What is Secondary Hypertension?

Secondary hypertension is high blood pressure caused by another medical condition. About 10-15% of all hypertension is believed to be "secondary". The most common "other medical conditions" are related to abnormal hormone levels or to narrowing of the arteries in the kidney (renal artery stenosis). Hormonal abnormalities that can cause hypertension include thyroid problems, Cushings syndrome, and pheochromocytoma. (Table 5).

When might your doctor suspect secondary hypertension? Additional testing to determine whether you have secondary hypertension might arise if you have high blood pressure but you:

- Had blood pressure consistently in normal range for many years prior to development of hypertension.
- Are experiencing rapidly increasing and out- of -control hypertension.
- Developed high blood pressure when you were less than 30-years old.
- Are not obese or overweight.
- Do not have a family history of primary hypertension.

It is important to determine whether you have secondary rather than primary hypertension since the treatment options could be drastically different.

Table 5. Common Causes of Secondary Hypertension

Condition	Abnormality	Prevalence (% of hypertensive patients)*	Characteristics in Addition to High Blood Pressure
Primary aldosteronism	Excess secretion of aldosterone by adrenal gland	8-10%	Low blood potassium, muscle weakness or cramping, excessive urination at night
Hypothyroidism	Reduced thyroid hormone secretion	1%	Low heart rate, cold intolerance, constipation, weight gain
Renal artery stenosis	Narrowing of arteries to the kidney due to plaque accumulation from atherosclerosis or to fibromuscular dysplasia	0.5-4%	Onset of hypertension without family history, often associated with "abdominal bruit" (a sound that can be heard by physician) and high blood renin
Cushing's syndrome	Excess cortisol production, sometimes due to tumor in pituitary or adrenal gland (rarely elsewhere)	less than 1%	Weight gain, thinning skin that bruises easily, "moon" face, stretch marks on abdomen/thighs; abnormal menstrual cycle
Pheochromocytoma	Tumor in adrenal gland that overproduces epinephrine	0.01-.1%	Highly variable blood pressure with sudden peaks that are often associated

	and norepinephrine (commonly known as adrenaline and noradrenaline)		with headache, palpitations, perspiration

Prevalence rates from reference 72— except renal artery stenosis from reference 52

First Discovery of PA

Most doctors practicing today were taught that PA, also called Conn's syndrome, is very rare, occurring in less than 1% of the population. PA was discovered by Dr. Jerome Conn in the 1950's. He had a 34-year-old patient with a group of symptoms, including high blood pressure that did not fit any of the known causes and was not cured by traditional medications for high blood pressure. Through evaluation of the patient and use of his medical knowledge, he determined that a hormone, aldosterone, was unusually high. He observed an adrenal tumor in a diagnostic image and went on to cure the patient through removal of the adrenal (adrenalectomy). He continued to study and publish findings on patients with high blood aldosterone over the next 20 years. Doctors trained after this discovery understood that high blood pressure of a small percent of the population might be caused by inappropriately high aldosterone. In other words, "aldosteronism" could be a cause of secondary hypertension.

As recently as the 1990's, most doctors believed PA to be very rare and only diagnosed in hypertensive patients who had frank hypokalemia (blood potassium concentration below the normal range, see Chapter 5). Since then, studies clarify that it is much more common than originally believed and is not always associated with hypokalemia.

How Many People Have PA?

Over the last 20 years, new estimates of the prevalence of PA have surfaced based on careful assessment of patients presenting with hypertension or of autopsies of patients after their death. The latest estimate is that about 8-10% of all individuals with hypertension have PA, and up to 20% of those with resistant hypertension have PA. For example, the Endocrine Society [28] estimates that about 10% of all hypertensive and 17-23% of resistant hypertensive patients have PA once the appropriate tests are performed. One of the studies supporting this estimate comes from an evaluation of over 1100 newly diagnosed hypertensive patients at 14 centers in Italy [65]. Each patient was further evaluated for PA using the diagnostic tests later described in this book (blood potassium, aldosterone-renin ratio, CT imaging, adrenal venous sampling, see Chapter 5). Using accepted criteria,

11.2% of these hypertensive patients had PA. Although various researchers and clinicians will argue about the specific proportion, the prevalence of PA is likely at least ten times above the less than 1% that many physicians were taught in their early medical training!

Let's convert this to numbers of actual people. According to the American Heart Association, in 2015 about 80 million people have hypertension in the US. If we use the estimate from the Endocrine Society that about 10% of these individuals have PA, this represents eight million people! Others have estimated the number of individuals with PA as at least 10 million [26]. How does this compare to other medical conditions? The CDC estimates that about 1.5 million people have rheumatoid arthritis, 1.1 million HIV, and around 1 million Parkinson's disease. These diseases are all much less common than the estimate for PA. To give more perspective, eight million is about the current population of New York City or the state of Virginia. Only 12 states have populations larger than eight million.

There are some assumptions used to come up with these estimates but even if this overestimates the number of people who have PA, none of the experts would dispute that there are millions of people with PA, many who are unaware they have it. Dr. John Funder estimates that about 1% of those with PA have been diagnosed [27], suggesting that about 80,000 people in the US are being treated for PA leaving over seven million people undiagnosed and inadequately or inappropriately treated.

Clearly this is a serious condition that is underestimated and under-diagnosed by many in the medical community. It affects many people, increasing their risk of disability and death. We need more education and focus on this condition.

Who Gets PA?

Most PA is diagnosed when patients are 30-60 years old. A small proportion of people are diagnosed as children; this is usually a genetic form of PA (covered in Chapter 6). There are no data to suggest the incidence is different in men compared to women, by race, or that lifestyle factors like diet and/or physical activity predict incidence. We don't know what personal factors are associated with development of PA. We are lacking large studies that can fully describe the characteristics of the typical PA patient.

Medical Consequences of PA

Hypertension was listed earlier as a risk factor for cardiovascular disease. However, the increase in risk for those with PA is several times higher than for those with the same degree of blood pressure elevation caused by primary hypertension. Evidence shows that the risk of stroke is four times, heart attack (myocardial infarction) is six times, and a specific heart arrhythmia (atrial fibrillation) is 12 times as likely to develop in those with PA compared to the same blood pressure in those without PA [54]. This is serious! It is imperative that PA patients are correctly diagnosed and treated to reduce their risk of these serious complications.

Chapter 4

WHAT IS THE ROLE OF ALDOSTERONE AND WHY DOES IT GO TERRIBLY WRONG?

What Does Aldosterone Normally Do?

Aldosterone is important enough that we could not survive without it. To understand the normal role of aldosterone, see Figure 3. In a nutshell, aldosterone is critical in helping us regulate the amount of water, sodium, and potassium we have in our bodies. Various chemicals and hormones work together with aldosterone to regulate body water and sodium (Table 6).

The kidney plays an important role in maintaining normal body fluid and minerals like sodium, potassium, and phosphate. Kidneys are made up of a million or more "filters" (called nephrons) that filter blood. Excess water and waste products move into the urine, but the kidney can send some minerals or water back into the blood, as needed. Normally, the kidney is adept at balancing the volume of urine and its contents for what you are consuming and what your body needs. If you have accumulated too much water or sodium, the kidney allows more water and sodium to be passed into the urine for excretion. Alternatively, if there is low blood flow in the kidney, this is sensed as a warning to increase movement of sodium and water from the urine into the blood.

Technical Discussion #1

The kidney's ability to balance water and minerals is controlled by various chemicals and hormones (see Table 6 and Figure 3). If, for example, you have lost a lot of water and sodium through sweating, you may be dehydrated and have a low blood volume. Your blood pressure could get drastically low resulting in less blood and oxygen getting to the brain causing dizziness with possible progression to unconsciousness.

To prevent the drop in blood pressure from going too far, a cascade of events take place in the body. First, the kidney will release a protein, renin, that activates angiotensinogen, that has been released from the liver, to create angiotensin I. An enzyme, Angiotensin Converting Enzyme (ACE), produced in the lungs and some other tissues, converts angiotensin I to angiotensin II. Angiotensin II is a powerful chemical that can cause constriction of the arteries and stimulate the adrenal gland to produce and secrete aldosterone. Aldosterone acts directly on the kidney to increase the reabsorption of water and sodium that passes through the kidney so that less sodium is lost in the urine. The increase in water and sodium retention will bring your blood volume back to normal, stop the release of renin, and break this cycle. Note that there is a feedback loop in that high aldosterone normally reduces production of renin in the kidney. This is the "shut off" signal to indicate that normalization of blood volume or sodium has occurred and relieves the need to reabsorb extra sodium and water.

Table 6. Definition of Factors in the Renin-Angiotensin-Aldosterone System

Term	Definition
RAAS	Renin, angiotensin, aldosterone system
Renin	Protein produced in the kidney in response to low kidney blood volume
Angiotensinogen	Protein produced in the liver
Angiotensin I	Produced from angiotensinogen when exposed to renin
Angiotensin II	Produced from angiotensin I by ACE; stimulates production of aldosterone
Angiotensin Converting Enzyme (ACE)	Enzyme expressed in the lung that converts angiotensin I to angiotensin II
Aldosterone	Hormone produced in adrenals in response to angiotensin II

Figure 3. Normal Renin- Angiotensin- Aldosterone System Responding to Low Blood Volume.

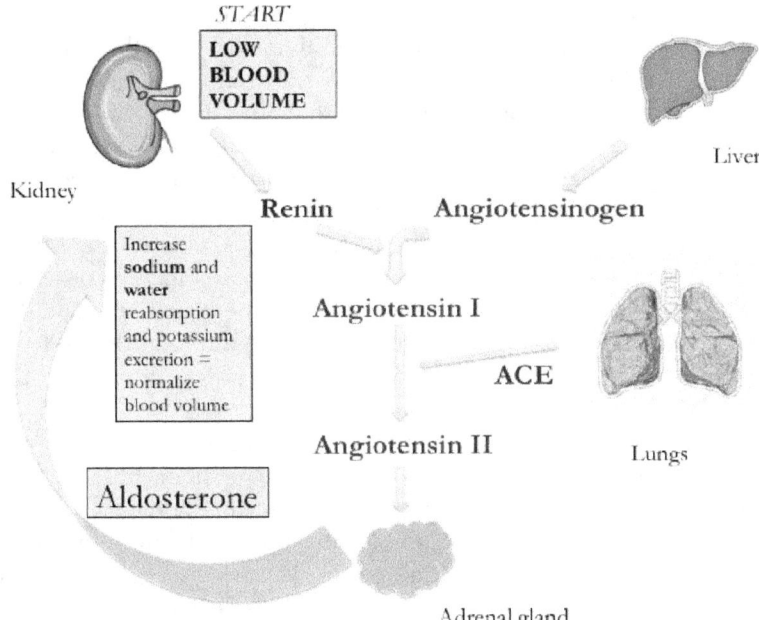

A variety of situations can trigger an increase in blood aldosterone, including:

- Low blood sodium
- Low blood volume
- High blood potassium
- High blood angiotensin II
- ACTH (a hormone put out by pituitary in times of stress)
- Posture (secretion is higher when standing than lying down)
- Hard exercise or emotional stress

End Technical Discussion #1

Why is Aldosterone Too High in PA and What Does This Do?

As described above, aldosterone is primarily produced by the adrenal glands. You have two adrenals, one just above each kidney. For most people, the secretion of aldosterone will be reduced once they have gotten their blood volume, sodium, and pressure to normal. However, in patients with PA, aldosterone is secreted in spite of the normal "turn off" signals (*e.g.* low renin). In some people, this occurs since a tumor (called an adenoma) in one of the adrenals ignores the normal signals and produces excessive aldosterone. In other people, the excess aldosterone is produced by both adrenals because of development of abnormal cells that overgrow (hyperplasia). The first type of PA is named APA (aldosterone-producing adenoma) while the second is called IHA (idiopathic hyperaldosteronism) due to abnormal cell growth (hyperplasia) on both adrenals—see more on this in Chapter 6. Note that neither of these conditions is cancer! It is possible to have a cancerous adrenal tumor, but it is rare (see Chapter 5).

When aldosterone is excessively high, the kidneys will reabsorb higher than usual amounts of sodium and water, creating an increase in blood volume. This high blood volume puts pressure on the blood vessel walls— thus hypertension develops. The higher blood pressure actually assists in reducing the excessive sodium since kidney blood flow increases urine sodium excretion.

Aldosterone also increases blood pressure through mechanisms beyond the kidney, including effects on the central nervous system, heart, and the blood vessels. In addition, aldosterone sensitizes the body to common stimulators of hypertension. For example, the body may overreact to an increase in hormones (such as angiotensin II, norepinephrine and/or epinephrine [49, 73]. It is interesting to note that although the effect of aldosterone on the kidney is likely the main way that this hormone causes hypertension, individuals who have end-stage renal disease and virtually no kidney function still become hypertensive when faced with high aldosterone levels [73]. So the kidney is only one organ and system affected by aldosterone.

What Causes the Adrenal Adenoma or Hyperplasia?

There is currently no satisfactory answer to explain why most people develop PA. Although a small proportion of PA has known genetic causes, most of PA is not thought to be predetermined at birth. Are there some characteristics or behaviors that increase your risk? Scientists do not know at this time. Hopefully, as more research is done, we will develop a list of risk factors (as we discussed earlier have been developed for cardiovascular disease) that will help us identify those at higher risk of developing PA. These "at-risk" individuals could be encouraged to take special precautions to prevent PA or to have regular testing. In the meantime, we have to improve our ability to identify PA among those people reporting to physicians with hypertension.

How Does PA Evolve?

PA does not start suddenly on one day. There is a progression of the disease that finally unveils itself through symptoms [33]. Early in the disease you might have vague symptoms—getting up extra times during the night to empty your bladder, headaches, fuzzy thinking—that could be dismissed as just part of aging. The excessive urination at night is your body's attempt to rid itself of the excess sodium and water that is accumulating. One way to increase loss of excessive body sodium is to increase the blood pressure and flow within the kidney. An increase in blood flow in the kidney, by itself, will increase urine sodium excretion in the urine and thus reduction of the excessive sodium. This explains the frequent urination symptom that often accompanies PA. However, if the excess aldosterone persists, your body will no longer be able to fully excrete the extra sodium and water. Thus blood pressure rises and sustained hypertension develops. This is usually the stage that brings a patient to a doctor. The longer someone goes without treatment, the more dramatic blood pressure problems will likely be.

Technical Discussion #2

Negative Effects of High Aldosterone beyond Blood Pressure

The fact that PA is associated with much higher risk of stroke and heart attack than the same blood pressure from primary hypertension reveals that all the negative effects of excessive aldosterone are not limited to its effect on blood pressure. In fact, many new research studies have been published to show that aldosterone has toxic effects on many organs in the body.

Heart

High blood pressure is known to cause impairment of heart anatomy and function. The level of damage with PA is beyond that caused by high blood pressure. There are receptors for aldosterone in heart cells. Stimulation of these receptors with aldosterone can induce enlargement and fibrosis of the heart [10]. This means that the heart gets thicker and stiffer and does not function as well as a pump. People with PA are about twice as likely to be diagnosed with left ventricular hypertrophy (LVH), thickening of the lower chamber of the heart, as those with the same blood pressure from primary hypertension. Since LVH increases risk of heart failure, this is a concern. Some heart changes, as detected by echocardiogram (uses ultrasound to measure the heart chamber dimensions as well as contraction) have been noted before high blood pressure develops.

Abnormalities of the heart contraction cycle are called arrhythmias. The cardiac fibrosis from PA mentioned in the previous paragraph can contribute to arrhythmias by disrupting the electrical coordination of heart contraction [32]. In addition, disturbance of sodium and potassium levels in the blood and cells can stimulate arrhythmias. The most common arrhythmia in PA is atrial fibrillation. As mentioned previously, the risk of atrial fibrillation is estimated to be 12 times higher for people with PA.

Kidney

The kidney has an intricate filtering system with delicate membranes that allow water and minerals to move across them. The kidneys help us adjust to excesses or deficiencies of water and electrolytes like sodium and potassium. An increase in blood pressure forces excess blood volume at a high pressure through the kidney (resulting in a high "glomerular filtration rate" in lab results). This high pressure can damage these delicate membranes, causing them to thickening and rendering them less effective. As with the heart, there is evidence that aldosterone causes fibrosis and kidney damage beyond that that would be expected due to high blood pressure alone [67]. Kidney damage is determined by signs including observation of protein in the urine, or with advanced disease, abnormally low glomerular filtration rate. When scientists injected aldosterone into rats, some proteins got forced through the kidney membranes into the urine (proteinuria) and the kidneys became sclerotic (rigid and less functional as a filter of blood) [9]. This supports that aldosterone can damage kidneys.

Brain, Nervous System, Behavior

High "sympathetic drive" is a hallmark of most hypertension. The sympathetic nervous system is the part of our nervous system that activates the "flight or flight" response. It revs up the heart, contracts blood vessels, and increases sweating. This is critical if you are in an emergency situation and need to escape from danger, but it can have negative consequences—including high blood pressure if it is repeated or becomes chronic. High sympathetic drive is thought to cause some of the medical issues in obese individuals and those with heart failure; aldosterone increases sympathetic drive [46].

Some of the symptoms mentioned by PA patients on Internet posts suggest high sympathetic drive as they use words such as "jittery", "anxiety", "acute alertness". An increase in sympathetic drive could contribute to difficulty sleeping and "obstructive sleep apnea." Sleep apnea means that the individual stops breathing sporadically at night. Often it is accompanied by snoring. Researchers at the University of Alabama found that plasma aldosterone concentration correlated to the magnitude of sleep apnea in patients with resistant hypertension [31] and that a medication that blocks aldosterone (spironolactone) reduced severity of sleep apnea [29]. This does not prove that aldosterone causes all sleep apnea but it suggests they can be connected.

Some individuals with PA complain of "fuzzy brain," depression, or high levels of anxiety. Clinicians hypothesize that this might be a consequence of low blood potassium or could be caused by elevated chemicals released due to inflammation caused by aldosterone.

> *Sometimes I would feel like my body was on autopilot, like I was going through the motions of life. I've not had the feeling on spiro[nolactone], only before treatment. (Shahall)*

Some PA patients complain of various negative psychological symptoms. A comparison of 23 PA patients to 23 primary hypertension patients demonstrated that PA patients were three times as likely to have diagnosed anxiety disorder and had higher scores on a stress evaluation tool than those with primary hypertension [68].

Dr. Stowasser, a PA expert from Australia [69], summarizes anecdotal information from hospital physicians and staff saying that, in general, PA patients appear angrier, more impatient and irritable than patients with primary hypertension. Obviously, it is not reasonable to ascribe these emotions solely to PA, but there are examples such as the case study he reported of a highly irritable, angry man who had dramatically reduced negative emotions during the days following removal of his adrenal that caused normalization of blood aldosterone and potassium.

This description prompted Dr. Stowasser to perform a study of the "quality of life (QOL)" of 43 PA patients. Responses showed that PA patients had lower quality of life for four of the eight domains of the survey instrument (physical functioning, role physical, general health, vitality) than reported for average Australians. Both surgical and medical (drug) treatment reduced the negative quality of life indicators. Surgical patients had a more rapid improvement such that they were similar to normal within three months; medically treated patients attained normal scores on all measures except for "vitality" by six months [69].

Some patients report dramatic improvement in psychological symptoms after appropriate treatment of their PA. One individual noted on the Internet that they were able to stop the psychiatric medications they had been prescribed for anxiety and rages when they were correctly treated for PA.

Why might PA patients report lower quality of life? There could be multiple reasons, including those unrelated to PA (*e.g.*, personal life stresses) but factors related to PA could include: response to low blood potassium, high blood aldosterone, drug side effects, inflammation-related chemicals (e.g. cytokines) induced by high aldosterone, sleep problems caused by sympathetic nervous system activation, or others we don't understand yet. Interestingly, rats injected with aldosterone exhibited anxiety-like behavior but if they were also given eplerenone (which combats effects of high aldosterone, see Chapter 7) with the aldosterone, the anxiety behavior was reversed [36]. This study supports a connection between high aldosterone and anxious behavior that can be prevented with appropriate medication.

Pancreas

The pancreas releases insulin in response to a rise in blood glucose that occurs after you eat a carbohydrate meal. Since continuously high blood glucose is damaging to cells, it is important to bring it down to normal levels. Insulin normally takes care of this by nudging glucose into your body cells for use or storage. Potassium is pulled into the cells along with glucose, which may contribute to a lower blood potassium level when insulin is high. When insulin release is impaired or insulin does not work as efficiently as it should, pre-diabetes and eventually diabetes develops.

Aldosterone inhibits insulin action and thus can worsen some abnormalities associated with diabetes such as vascular dysfunction [7]. Aldosterone reduces pancreatic release of insulin in response to blood glucose and reduces insulin sensitivity in muscle and fat tissue [48]. Thus high blood aldosterone apparently increases the risk of developing insulin resistance and can worsen health status in those with diabetes.

Bone

Although there is not much research on the connection between aldosterone and bone, it is known that elevated aldosterone is associated with higher blood concentration of parathyroid hormone (PTH), a critical hormone controlling blood calcium [70]. PTH increases the loss of calcium from bones into the blood. As a consequence, the amount of calcium in urine may increase and add to the risk of kidney stones. Clinical cases of individuals with PA and recurrent kidney stones that resolved when they were treated for PA have been published in the medical literature [66].

About 30% of patients with PA have been measured as having higher PTH than those with the same blood pressure from primary hypertension. The net effect could be an increased loss of calcium and magnesium from the bone with possible impact on bone calcium and strength over time. One recent study [60] observed higher urinary calcium, higher blood PTH, and a higher prevalence of osteoporosis or osteopenia (low bone mineral) in PA. Although this suggests that patients with untreated PA could be at higher risk of bone fracture in PA, this would require longer-term studies to verify.

End Technical Discussion #2

Chapter 5

DIAGNOSING PA

What Kind of Doctor is Best to Diagnose and Treat PA?

There are some family doctors who may be knowledgeable about PA. However, that was not my experience. If you do not believe you are getting care from someone who understands and has experience with PA, I suggest you explore working with a more specialized doctor. There are "hypertension specialists" who should be more knowledgeable about this condition and the appropriate tests or treatments. There are websites that you can use to search for a hypertension specialist near you—go to the American Society of Hypertension website (http://www.ash-us.org). Click on "Hypertension Specialists Directory" and search by city, state, or country.

Ideally, I believe working with an endocrinologist who specializes in hypertension would provide the best insights and training to help someone with PA. However, you may not be able to find such a person locally. Some patients work with nephrologists (kidney specialists), especially if there is some indication of kidney impairment or damage (*e.g.* low glomerular filtration rate, excretion of protein in the urine).

> *I went 2 years with uncontrollable high blood pressure as my PC [primary care] doctor tried every combination of blood pressure drugs out there. It wasn't until my potassium level dropped so far it put my heart into tachycardia (which led to an ablation and insertion of a pacemaker) and I changed PC doctors that I was referred*

to Endocrinology because my new PC knew to test for aldosterone. Once I met with the Endo [endocrinologist] in January things went super fast. CT scan in January, AVS in February, and left adrenalectomy on March 6th. Getting the right doctors makes all of the difference. (Freeste)

Be persistent if you have questions about your treatment or diagnosis. If your persistence is greeted by irritation or a demeaning response, consider finding another doctor. See this comment:

I sure wish the doctors at the blood pressure clinic at ……. Medical had thought to give me a trial dose of Spiro[nolactone]. God knows they had me taking about everything else. My diagnosis would have been made by that simple test. Instead they kept doubling down on my 5 virtually useless bp meds. Then when I went in with a bp of 224/114, they let me walk out of there. (Dianne)

Patients Diagnosing Themselves

Searching on the Internet, you will find many tragic stories of people who suffered for years with hypertension and related ailments without a correct diagnosis and treatment. Some medical personnel label patients "crazy" or "noncompliant" as they believe they've given a treatment that "should" work. Women, especially, describe being told that their problems are psychological and relate to being a high-strung female. I was told by one doctor to "take a valium or a glass of wine" to calm down and I'd be fine. I knew my newly wildly erratic and super-elevated blood pressures were not because of my mental health.

Some patients have discovered information about PA on their own using the Internet and are amazed to find that their symptoms and progression match this condition. Here are examples of posts from individuals who had high blood pressure for many years before realizing this was due to PA:

I googled "primary hyperaldosteronism" and began reading what I could find. That led me to the NORD (National Organization for Rare Diseases) site. On that site I found a bunch of stories of people who had all the same symptoms I had, many of which I had never even connected to my condition. I started crying as I read them.

I wasn't nuts and didn't have Middle-Age Women's Syndrome. I was sick. (Dianne)

I went home and started Googling and discovered that adrenalomas plus low K [potassium] plus peeing a lot and increased thirst (which I also had) = PA. I was scheduled for another BP check at my primary doc's so I brought the CT scan info and all the PA info I found with me. She said that it was highly unlikely that I had PA, because "it's rare", and besides, my K [potassium] was fine. I asked to see that most recent K lab report -- the one that her office had told me was normal. It was 3.4 and labeled "Low"!!!!!!! (Joyce)

Some people do not know they have PA until they have a medical test for some other reason that reveals evidence of PA. See the following example posted on the Internet:

In 2002, at age 44, while in the hospital for a hysterectomy due to fibroids, I was told by the anesthesiologist who reviewed my pre-surgery labs that my potassium was low. I had no idea, and I don't think I was having symptoms of low potassium. When I think back, I remember having a lot of bad headaches, but this was a time of much stress and anxiety....... The only other PA symptom that jumps out at me in hindsight is that I was getting up several times a night to pee, but thought that was normal. (Joyce)

Other individuals may have a suspicious nodule discovered on an abdominal CT scan done for a reason such as abdominal pain. Finally, some may have been treated with a mineralocorticoid drug for another reason (*e.g.*, acne) and noticed unexpected improvements in their high blood pressure.

Symptoms

Symptoms are unusual feelings or function you experience that may give a clue to diagnosing a medical condition. Signs are conditions that someone else observes, *e.g.*, heavy sweating, red face.

Common symptoms in individuals who are later diagnosed with PA

include:
- Fatigue
- Headache
- Muscle weakness or cramps
- Numbness
- Polyuria (excessive urination, especially at night)
- Polydipsia (excessive thirst)

Not every patient experiences all of these symptoms but usually at least several. Additional symptoms mentioned by some people with PA include:
- Excessive sweating
- Constipation
- Tingling
- Panic/anxiety attacks
- Flank pain/discomfort

None of these symptoms is confined to PA so the doctor needs to do additional testing to determine the cause of these complaints that should be considered a warning that something is wrong.

High blood pressure is a typical reason that patients eventually diagnosed with PA initially seek medical care. High blood pressure from any cause can result in headaches, ringing in ears, and similar symptoms. However, most patients don't notice any symptoms of high blood pressure, and it might only be discovered incidentally during routine testing of blood pressure (as in my case).

Blood Potassium

After finding high blood pressure, the doctor will likely ask for a blood sample analysis. Most routine blood analyses include serum potassium. If serum potassium is below the normal range – usually considered below 3.5 mmol/L (millimoles per liter), this increases your likelihood of having PA. When you look at your blood test results, the units for potassium might be given in mmol/L or meq/L (milliequivalents per liter)— these can be used interchangeably for potassium. The doctor should consider that this could be PA and call for additional testing since low serum potassium with high blood pressure is a hallmark of PA.

You might still have PA even if your blood potassium is in the normal range. Although many doctors learned that low potassium (called hypokalemia) is a requirement for PA, we now know that is not true. In fact, the majority of people with PA have serum potassium on the lower end of the normal range so do not have hypokalemia. The Endocrine

Society states that only 9-37% of PA patients have hypokalemia [28]. In general, symptom severity tends to be higher if the patient is hypokalemic.

Most of our body potassium (chemical symbol, "K") is inside cells, but some is within the blood stream. A reduction in blood potassium is a red flag that a diagnosis of PA should be considered. Normal blood potassium ranges between 3.5 and 5.0 mmol/L. Low blood potassium, hypokalemia, is a problem since this can trigger muscle spasms and even paralysis. Blood potassium is typically lower in PA patients, partly because aldosterone stimulates excretion of potassium in exchange for the sodium reabsorbed in the kidney. However, there is also evidence that there is an increase in movement of potassium out of blood into cells as another contributor to hypokalemia.

Table 7. Adult Blood Potassium Interpretation

Category	Concentration (mmol/L or meq/L)
Low	Less than 3.5
Normal	3.5-5
Mildly elevated	5.1-6.0
Moderately elevated	6.1-7
Severely elevated	Greater than 7

Note that normal values can vary by laboratory. Use the ranges provided by the lab analyzing the blood sample.

It is important to take the blood sample correctly when measuring blood potassium. Ideally, it is recommended that blood be withdrawn with use of a tourniquet for only a brief time to locate a vein, and that cells are separated from the plasma within 30 minutes of collection. Repeatedly making a fist to forcing blood into the tube, leaving a tourniquet on too long, or leaving the blood too long with the red blood cells can increase the outflow of potassium from cells, making the sample reading incorrectly higher than your actual blood potassium. If the plasma or serum appears red after it has been spun in the centrifuge (it should be a straw yellow color), the sample is not useful for potassium since this indicates break up of red blood cells (hemolysis) that will cause an inappropriately high potassium reading.

So based on the modest percentage of PA patients who present with hypokalemia and the frequent incorrect blood withdrawal procedure, it is probable that a simple measurement of blood potassium will not clarify whether you have PA. Depending on your medical history, the doctor might believe that a workup for PA is not indicated and might perform a set of tests to rule out other causes of secondary hypertension (see Table 4) such as pheochromocytoma or renal artery stenosis. In my case, my serum potassium was on the low end of normal but did not attract the attention of my doctor since it was not technically an "abnormal" value.

If your doctor suspects PA or eliminates other causes of hypertension he or she may choose to do more sophisticated tests for PA. The Endocrine Society [28] recommends that doctors use any of the following criteria to suspect and further test for PA:

- A blood pressure verified as 160/100 mm or greater.
- The individual is on at least three medications without achieving his/her blood pressure target.
- Hypokalemia (low blood potassium, usually considered less than 3.5 mmol/L).
- Hypertension with an adrenal mass or growth (*e.g.,* discovered via CT or other imaging).
- Hypertension with family history of early onset hypertension or stroke before 40 years of age.
- Patients with a first-degree relative (*e.g.,* father/mother, sibling, offspring) with PA.

A minority of experts believe screening should be performed on more people—all those newly diagnosed with hypertension—in order to catch the many individuals with PA who may be missed. Although this approach would be costly, the reduction in costs due to prevention of serious and expensive-to-treat medical conditions such as heart failure, kidney failure, or stroke could theoretically offset this.

Aldosterone/Renin Ratio (ARR)

A screening test that should be performed to determine if you have PA is measurement of two chemicals, aldosterone and renin, in the blood. Plasma aldosterone concentration (PAC) is given in units of ng/dl (nanograms per deciliter) while plasma renin activity (PRA) has units of ng/ml/h (nanogram per milliliter per hour) (Table 8). Note that sometimes aldosterone is given on the laboratory report in pg/ml (picograms per milliliter) units. One pg/ml is equal to 0.1 ng/dl. So, dividing the value for aldosterone in pg/ml by 10 would convert it to ng/dl. Although this discussion of units seems complicated and unnecessary, it may be useful if blood values are given to you with a non-typical unit and you want to determine whether it is beyond the normal range.

These measures are more expensive than the routine blood panel that includes serum potassium but should be available from most labs. There is no strict cut-off for this ratio, but values of 20-40 or higher are often used to define PA—the Endocrine Society [28] suggests 30 as the minimum ratio to indicate likelihood of PA. In other words, if your aldosterone was 25 ng/dl and renin was 0.5 ng/ml/h, the ratio is 50 (25 divided by 0.5). Some experts require that, in addition to the ARR, the aldosterone concentration be at least 15 ng/dl to diagnose PA. Note that it is important to have the aldosterone and renin in the correct units before you calculate the ratio and put them in context with the normal values provided by the laboratory doing the analysis.

The Endocrine Society [28] recommends that patients with a high ARR undergo additional testing to confirm the diagnosis of PA before initiating medication treatment. Treatment at this point with PA medications is appropriate only if the patient cannot or does not want to consider surgery as a possible treatment (see below), as eligibility for surgery would require additional testing.

Table 8. Definitions of Abbreviations for Blood Screening PA

ARR	Aldosterone/renin ratio
PAC	Plasma aldosterone concentration
PRA	Plasma renin activity

The specific guidelines for taking the blood sample for the aldosterone to renin ratio include that the sample be taken in the morning after being awake for several hours and that the patient should be seated rather than lying down. (Aldosterone concentration will usually be highest in mid-morning compared to afternoon) The patient should have been eating a diet unrestricted in salt prior to this test (Table 9). A low sodium diet could cause an artificially affect the ARR and mask the diagnosis. In addition, if serum potassium were observed to be low in the earlier routine blood panel, this should be normalized with potassium supplements prior to the evaluation of ARR.

One challenge in getting accurate aldosterone and renin values is that like most hormones, aldosterone varies in concentration over the day. So, one "normal" assessment does not exclude PA. A second challenge to our confidence in the test results may be interference from drugs that may impact the ARR. The Endocrine Society [28] recommends that aldosterone antagonists (eplerenone, spironolactone), amiloride, and potassium-losing diuretics (e.g. HCTZ) be withdrawn at least four weeks before the ARR test. If the results are ambiguous, other drugs such as beta-adrenergic blockers, ARB, ACEi, calcium channel blockers may also be withdrawn, using substitution with other hypertensive drugs that are not thought to substantially affect the ARR (*e.g.,* verapamil, hydralazine, doxazosin).

Figure 4. Diagnostic Tests for PA

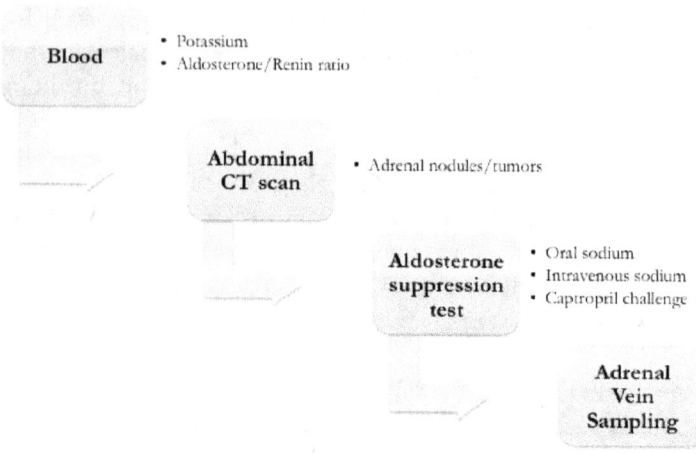

Withdrawal of hypertensive drugs may be dangerous for some patients. One study of patients with PA reported that withdrawal of hypertensive drugs and substitution with others was only possible in about half of their patients [21]. Some patients experienced extreme increases in blood pressure or heart rhythm abnormalities that required hospitalization or special treatment. The physician will decide on your personal risk for changing medications and will determine the best course of action.

What do you do if you are already on an aldosterone antagonist (eplerenone, spironolactone)? The recommendation is that these medications be stopped for at least 4-6 weeks before testing the ARR. Personally, I have been unwilling to do this since these drugs were so effective for me. Four or more weeks is a long time, in my mind, to be without drugs that successfully treat my illness. Thus I am still without a measurement of my ARR. At least some evidence suggests that the ARR is valid without stopping all hypertensive medications [30]. I will continue to watch for developments in the options for medication cessation for the ARR test.

Table 9. Preparation for Aldosterone/Renin Ratio (ARR) Test

Time period	Instructions
4-6 weeks before test	Withdraw from medications that could interfere with ARR
Several weeks before test	Correct low blood potassium with supplements.
The week before test	Eat a liberal sodium diet before test
The day of test	Collect blood sample mid-morning after patient has been awake for at least 2 hours
	Collect blood after patient has been seated for 5-15 minutes without substantial fist clenching; separate red blood cells within 30 minutes

Aldosterone Suppression Tests

If the ARR is higher than the recommended cut-off level, the Endocrine Society [28] recommends performance of any one of several types of aldosterone suppression tests (Figure 4). The goal of these tests is to see if the adrenals reduce their production and release of aldosterone in response to a normal "turn-off" signal—high blood sodium. Why is this necessary in addition to the ARR test? ARR is a "sensitive" but not a "specific" test. This means that ARR will be positive in some patients who ultimately do not have PA. In order to confirm the presence of PA, one of the aldosterone suppression tests is necessary (Figure 4).

Sodium loading is achieved either through three days of a high salt diet or through 4- hours of continuous injection of sodium through a tube placed in a blood vessel. In individuals without PA, aldosterone levels should fall to very low values after either the oral or the injected sodium challenge tests. The Endocrine Society [28] considers post-sodium loading aldosterone normal if less than 5 ng/dl, borderline if 5-10, and indicative of PA if greater than 10.

Here is an excerpt from the description of doing the oral-sodium-loading test by JaneRay1940 from her blog:

Some people can do this and feel just fine. Others will retain water, which will lead to all sorts of icky things like headaches, bloating, nausea, elevated blood pressure, heart palpitations, and so forth. I already know that I'll fall into that latter group – I can barely eat restaurant food without getting those symptoms thanks to all the salt most restaurants use.

A captropril challenge test might be your doctor's choice after the ARR instead of an oral or injected sodium test. The captropril test lasts several hours and involves orally ingesting captopril with blood measurements for renin, aldosterone and cortisol at baseline, at one and two hours after ingestion. Normally, aldosterone concentrations will be reduced at least 30% by the captropril ingestion. Aldosterone remains high in patients with PA.

Again, at this step a doctor and patient may decide he/she has enough information to medically treat the PA patient who does not want to consider a surgical option. However, if the patient and doctor want to know if there is a problem with only one or both adrenals, two other tests will be valuable in confirming the diagnosis.

CT Imaging

The Endocrine Society [28] recommends that all patients with PA undergo abdominal CT imaging (or MRI) to determine if a tumor or nodule is observed in either adrenal. This can provide evidence for surgical eligibility if only one adrenal is affected, and the test can also usually exclude adrenal cancer. Adrenal cancer is rare but obviously something you'd want to know about. CT scans can typically detect cancerous tumors that tend to be large (3 cm or more).

The CT uses x-rays to get cross-sectional images of your abdomen. The organs are viewed to look for abnormalities of anatomy or presence of tumors. My experience with this test was that it did not cause a high degree of discomfort but did cause some anxiety since I was given little advanced description. I recommend reading about the procedure on the Internet if your medical team does not fully explain the procedure. For me, it involved consuming a large volume (maybe a liter) of a sugary beverage over 40-60 minutes after arriving with an empty stomach. This is the "contrast" fluid that will help them visualize your digestive tract in the image.

After I had consumed most of the liquid, they had me go a room to lie on a narrow table. The nurse inserted an IV in my arm just prior to the imaging—this allows another contrast fluid to be injected during the scan to illuminate the blood vessels in the image. I was asked to put my arms above my head, be still, and hold my breath as the scanner passed over my body within a few seconds. I felt a warm sensation when the dye was injected into my IV. I did not experience any negative effects of the contrast or the IV. However, some people have a bad reaction to the contrast dye. Let your doctor know if you have had any negative reactions to contrast in the past or if you experience any unusual symptom during the procedure or afterwards. Although no one told me, I have read that it is a good idea to drink a lot of fluids after the procedure to accelerate excretion of the contrast dye.

Sometimes an unusual adrenal is noted when you have a CT scan performed for some other reason, such as abdominal pain. This is sometimes called an incidentaloma since it is an incidental finding.

It is important to realize that abdominal CT is only accurate in diagnosis of PA in about 53% of patients [28]. So lack of observation of an adrenal nodule/tumor does not rule out PA. The procedure also carries risk since there is radiation exposure. If the doctor/patient wants to exclude cancer, CT imaging is the way to do it. However, doctors will rarely rely on imaging alone to determine if one or two adrenals are involved in PA. One study of 35 PA patients reported that CT scans using the latest technology accurately matched adrenal vein blood sampling (AVS), the gold standard for PA diagnosis and lateralization (see below), in only about 66% of the cases [63].

Here is interesting evidence that one should not rely completely on the CT scan results:

> *I would never, ever get an adrenalectomy without an AVS as my CT scan indicated an adrenal bump on my right adrenal gland and not on my left. The AVS gave opposite results of what they were expecting. If I had gone off the CT scan, they would have taken out the wrong gland and I would still be so sick. (Dana)*

Adrenal Vein Sampling (AVS)

This procedure measures how much aldosterone each adrenal is secreting into the blood stream. It is typically considered essential for individuals who would consider surgery if the PA is found to be only from one adrenal. The procedure is performed by an interventional radiologist who threads a thin tube through blood vessels in your groin to the adrenal gland. Blood samples are collected as blood leaves each adrenal to detect if one or both of the glands is secreting excessive aldosterone.

This is a costly and highly technical procedure that is only performed in a modest number of hospitals, largely within academic medical centers. There is a relatively high failure rate, meaning that the results could be inconclusive. Usually "failure" is because of the technical difficulty getting the catheter to the correct location for blood samples. In this case, they cannot interpret the results and may decide to repeat the test. Failure more often happens on the right side since the anatomy of the vessels is more difficult to navigate.

In addition to having a high failure rate, there are risks that could be serious, such as adrenal vein rupture, infarction (blocked artery), thrombosis (blood clot leading to stroke). These risks are quite rare at most experienced centers. Of course, you will want to inquire about costs and insurance coverage as it can be an expensive procedure.

My suggestion is that if you decide to have this procedure, search for a center/hospital that has regular weekly experience using this technique. Similarly, care should be taken to select an endocrinologist experienced in interpretation of AVS results.

Most people describe the AVS as less painful and scary than they anticipated. I have not had AVS but provide below the description from individuals who posted their experiences on-line:

I had two AVS procedures. You will be awake but relaxed during the procedure. You will be able to feel some sensation but no pain. They will ask occasionally if you feel any hot sensations. I didn't. The hardest part for me was laying flat for the 4 hours afterwards to heal so you don't bleed out of the entry sight. They will give you medicine to sleep some of the time away. Take a book or magazine. I didn't have a room with a TV. You will have a little mark on each side of your groin. They don't hurt. You may get bruising the next day. Mine was pretty severe. It took 2 weeks to go away. AVS is pretty painless. The only good advice I have for you is to go to the bathroom before you leave the hospital to make sure your incisions don't bleed. (Dana)

The AVS was no big deal for me. Most get a little anxious but often report the worst part was laying flat on their back for two hours after the procedure! At NIH I had an attendant standing beside each hip, the IR [interventional radiologist] was seated on my right around waist level and a nurse was position by my head and explained everything that was going on..... After the procedure they will apply pressure in your groin area where they inserted the needles, this may take half an hour or so. Then they wheeled me back to my room and I had to lay flat on my back for two hours with a nurse checking my groin area often. I flew home the next day unattended. (John)

Soreness is also expected, and mine began 3 hours later. I felt pain in places I didn't expect- like my arms and lower legs. The pain was overwhelming in my groin area. Severe bruising started the next day and is expected, but it's important to make sure it's soft, not hard. As well, check your bandage for excessive bleeding. (JaneRay1040)

Based on our earlier estimate that there could be 8 million people in the US with PA, most unaware and inadequately treated, our limited capacity for performing AVS could be quickly overwhelmed if we were able to improve our screening for this condition. So, there is interest in developing alternative techniques to lateralize PA (decide whether it is on one adrenal or both). For example, I have read studies using a PET (positron emission tomography) scan combined with abdominal CT scan. Other research groups have focused on combining the results of other tests into a score that could predict eligibility for surgery [26]. However, these new procedures are experimental and not ready for widespread diagnostic use at this time. Development of a non-invasive test to lateralize PA would be a major breakthrough and may happen in the future.

Chapter 6

TYPES OF PA

Although all PA is a problem of too much aldosterone, this can arise for a variety of reasons.

Idiopathic Hyperaldosteronism (IHA)

A common cause of too much aldosterone is adrenal hyperplasia, estimated to be about 60% of PA. This is most often an issue in both adrenals and is caused by excessive growth of cells in the gland that produce aldosterone. Why do they overgrow? No one knows at this time, but I am sure more will be revealed as additional research accumulates. I am curious whether there is any effect of things like diet (*e.g.,* sodium intake), repeated dehydration (like that occurring with exercise), or stress since these conditions normally stimulate aldosterone synthesis. I hope to find research on this topic that I will post on my PA website.

Aldosterone-Producing Adenoma (APA)

The second most common cause of excessive aldosterone (~40% of PA) is development of adenomas, small noncancerous tumors that produce aldosterone. These adenomas are most often in one adrenal.

Patients with APA are often diagnosed earlier than IHA since their symptoms can be more severe with lower blood potassium and higher blood pressure. However, without clear evidence from AVS, it is not possible to definitively distinguish between APA and IHA.

A reason you may want to know the type of PA you have is in order to determine whether you would be eligible for surgery. The medical treatment (drug and diet, see below) is the same regardless of having IHA or APA, but if you have APA, you could be a candidate for surgical removal of the one abnormal gland. The next section will discuss this in more detail.

Technical Discussion #3

Genetic PA

Currently, the thinking is that genetically caused PA accounts for only about 1-5% of the diagnosed PA. This means that the individual was born with a mutation in their DNA that caused development of PA; they could pass it onto their children. The genetic subtypes identified at this time include:

FH-I (also called GRA for glucocorticoid-remediable aldosteronism)

Patients with FH-1 PA have early childhood onset (younger than age 20), severe hypertension, propensity to cerebrovascular accidents (strokes) and suppression of aldosterone secretion with glucocorticoid drugs such as dexamethasone. Abnormalities of two enzymes, aldosterone synthase and 11-beta-hydroxylase, increasing aldosterone and cortisol synthesis, respectively, are involved. In this type of PA, the synthesis of aldosterone is more controlled by the pituitary hormone, ACTH, than by the normal controller, angiotensin II. Estimates are that less than 1% of PA patients have the FH-I genetic mutation.

FH-II

This PA usually develops in adulthood and is more common than FH-I. It is suspected when at least two members of the family have PA where the aldosterone does not reduce when dexamethasone (a drug that normally reduces ACTH and aldosterone) is administered. The specific mutation causing FH-II is not known. FH-II is responsible for 1-6% of PA.

FH- III

Children (younger than 18 years) with a mutation of their potassium channel—opening in the cell membrane that controls movement of potassium into or out of the cell—with large adrenals may have this type of PA. Most of these individuals have severe hypertension and hypokalemia at an early age. The hyperplasia is present in both adrenals. The mutations responsible for FH-III are in the KCNJ5 gene encoding the potassium channel GIRK4. Less than 1% of PA patients are thought to have FH-III.

These sub-types of PA may be treated differently than other types of PA. For example, FH-1 is usually treated with a glucocorticoid drug such as dexamethasone or prednisone. This will reduce the pituitary production of ACTH and then reduce the stimulation of aldosterone production at the adrenal gland.

Why would you want to know if you have a genetically related PA? You would want to alert your family so that they might consider being evaluated or consider this as part of your decision on having children. Diagnosis with one of these genetically- related PA types requires analysis of your DNA. Although this is not a painful test—usually a small blood sample is enough—it is not routinely done most places, is usually very expensive, and is not likely covered by your insurance company. This would likely only be done if they have very high suspicion that you could have a genetically caused type of PA that may require specific treatment. This might be suggested if two or more members of your family appear to have PA or if your PA was diagnosed when you were a child.

Somatic Mutations

Medical researchers are also looking into somatic mutations as a cause of PA. Somatic mutations are mutations of DNA that did not exist when you were born but developed later, possibly from environmental stresses. These mutations are relevant only for you and are not passed onto your children. Somatic mutations of membrane channels and enzymes that control the movement of sodium and potassium across cell membranes have been identified in PA patients [76]. A recent medical review paper estimated that more than half of APA is due to a somatic mutation in the DNA that codes for proteins (abbreviated by the acronyms, KCNJ5, ATP1A1, ATP2B3, CACNAID) [76].

Table 10. Definition of Types of DNA Mutations

Genetic mutation	Mutation of the DNA that exists at birth, may pass onto children
Somatic mutation	Mutation of the DNA that occurs after birth, does not pass onto children

Secondary Aldosteronism

High blood aldosterone can be caused by reasons that do not involve abnormal adrenal cells but is instead a normal reaction to low blood sodium or volume. For example, if you have a condition that causes excessive kidney excretion of sodium via the urine (e.g. Gitelman syndrome), your body will react to restore sodium by releasing more aldosterone to increase reabsorption of sodium and water. Another example, of secondary aldosteronism is renal artery stenosis. When renal arteries are reduced in diameter because of atherosclerosis, the kidney perceives this as low blood volume and reacts by stimulating the production of more renin, and as a consequence, aldosterone (see Figure 3). In these cases, the high aldosterone is "secondary" to the first problem.

End Technical Discussion #3

❖

Chapter 7

SURGICAL AND MEDICAL TREATMENTS FOR PA

The last section should have convinced you that it is essential to get treatment for PA as soon as possible to avoid some of the negative consequences of high aldosterone. Luckily, there is evidence that treating PA, either through medications or surgery, reduces your long-term risk of complications such as stroke, arrhythmia, heart attack, and kidney deterioration. In fact, there is evidence that treatment reverses many of the complications described in Chapter 4.

One of the first studies to compare surgery to medication treatment [8] followed 54 patients with PA and 323 with primary hypertension. About half of the PA patients were treated with medication and the other half with surgery. They were followed over seven years to determine cardiovascular outcomes including heart attack, stroke, bypass surgery, and arrhythmias. Initially, patients with PA had 4.6 times the likelihood of cardiovascular events than patients with similar blood pressure from primary hypertension. By the follow-up point, a similar proportion (approximately 18%) of patients with PA or with primary hypertension had cardiovascular events, meaning that the extra risk of PA above that of primary hypertension was eliminated with treatment. In addition, the researchers observed no difference in this risk improvement whether the PA patients had been treated with medications or surgery.

An example of evidence for the benefit of treatment is the elimination or reduction of excessive thickening of the left side of the heart (left ventricular hypertrophy) in PA patients after a year or more of treatment. This can be observed by doing an echocardiogram before and after treatment.

Surgery

If you are found to have excess aldosterone production from only one adrenal, you may be offered surgical treatment. This is usually done laparoscopically which means that the surgeon inserts a tube to do the surgery rather than through a larger incision. Laparoscopic surgery is considered less risky and causes less scar formation than surgery with an incision. The surgeon will usually remove the entire adrenal gland although in some European countries, clinicians will attempt to remove only the tumor and leave part of the adrenal gland.

Care should be taken in selecting an endocrine surgeon to perform adrenalectomy. The following is taken from an NIH website (http://www.nichd.nih.gov/health/topics/adrenalgland/conditioninfo/pages/faqs.aspx) answering "How do I find an experienced adrenal surgeon?":

> *Make sure that the surgeon you choose is experienced. This means that he or she performs at least 20 adrenal operations a year. Be sure to ask surgeons how many operations they perform each year and what their complication rates are. Your endocrinologist or primary care team should be able to recommend good surgeons in your geographic area. For more information, visit the American Association of Endocrine Surgeons patient education website at http://endocrinediseases.org.*

Should you have the surgery if offered? The answer is complicated and different for each individual. You, with your doctor, should weigh the decision based on issues like severity of your condition, risk of complications, likelihood of resolution of your symptoms, and whether you are getting effective and low side-effect improvement with diet and medications. Are you willing to diligently take the mediations/adhere to dietary limitations—likely for your lifetime? The information below might help you make a decision on surgery verses medicine.

Likelihood of Improvement Post- Surgery

Data collected on individuals who had adrenalectomy (removal of one adrenal) show that about 50-70% are "cured" meaning they no longer need to take medications or restrict their diet to maintain normal aldosterone and blood pressure levels. So 30-50% continue to need some medications—usually at reduced doses—and with dietary effort. How can you tell which one you will be? It is not possible to know with certainty, but usually patients who have had hypertension a longer time are more likely to still need some medications.

If you are one of those who is "cured," you no longer need to restrict your dietary sodium as diligently as before. However, as a nutritionist, I feel it important to suggest that you consider following a healthy diet that includes no more than 2300 mg sodium (see Chapter 8), the amount recommended for all adults by the Federal dietary guidelines.

Many people who have had adrenalectomy report amazingly improved life, usually very quickly after the surgery. One person noted that they had "tons of energy, no more naps, very calm, no brain fog, memory is better, pains are less, hair is growing faster and is healthier, no more late day eye blurriness, hands." Other patients described their experience:

> *It's been almost a year since my adrenalectomy and being drug free. It's amazing how so many "symptoms" disappeared when I stopped taking all those medications. I was on 6 different blood pressure pills a day and 2 Potassium supplements and my blood pressure was still really high. (Freeste)*

> *I started to get energy bursts within one and a half week. I can't begin to explain my euphoria over this. Another good, though odd, change was sweating-- I didn't sweat the last 2 years, and now I perspire quite easily. There is a now a normal frequency of nightly bathroom visits-- instead of 4-5 times, I'm back to my one nocturnal trip. The migraines are gone, helleujah. Major Bonus: I no longer take 5 medications, which were stopped immediately post-surgery. (C.A. Langrall from her blogspot site)*

Although extremely rare, it is possible that you will develop PA in your remaining adrenal after an adrenalectomy. In that case, they will treat you with medication and diet since it is very difficult to continue without any adrenal gland as we rely on some of the other hormones the adrenal produces (*e.g.* epinephrine, cortisol).

Complications

Like any surgery, there can be complications, *e.g.*, post operative bleeding, infection, hernia at incision. The complication rate is relatively low (less than 1%) with adrenalectomy done laparoscopically. A review of 43 scientific articles reporting outcomes of adrenalectomy for PA; the average complication rate for 1056 patients was 4.7% [57]

Recovery after Adrenalectomy

Spironolactone or eplerenone are typically discontinued after the surgery; the doctor will decide whether other blood pressure medications are withdrawn or reduced based on your blood pressure response.

Rarely, patients can experience a short-term period of unusually low aldosterone following adrenalectomy. The remaining adrenal may have gotten used to not producing aldosterone since the other released so much. It might take time for it to take on its role of producing normal levels of this hormone. In the meantime, those who experience this condition may have very low blood pressure and dizziness. A clinical concern can develop if this continues since low aldosterone can lead to low blood sodium (hyponatremia) and high blood potassium (hyperkalemia)—both can be serious. A simple blood test can inform the doctor if this is something he/she needs to attend to. Blood potassium will be typically measured closely for the first week.

My understanding of what you might experience after adrenalectomy comes from what I have read from patients who have undergone this surgery. Most individuals report some pain that is typically manageable with short-term use of oral pain relievers. The pain relievers can cause their own set of side effects such as constipation, so use only as much as you need. One of the most frequently mentioned complaints is gas pressure from the introduction of gas into the body cavity that occurs during the procedure. This resolves over time, but you may find certain positions more comfortable than others. Return to modest activities, including driving, is often allowed within a few days, but your doctor will let you know what he/she recommends.

> *Of course there was some pain, which was managed with painkillers. For me, the pain was mainly in my midsection, and it hurt more standing and walking. It wasn't too bad after about 5 days. Some other people get pain in the shoulder region. The incisions did not hurt me much, except when laying on the side where the incisions were made. I had to sleep on one side and my back for a while. Painkillers can cause constipation, so I cut back on them as soon as I could. I was able to drive short distances within three days. I also avoided lifting anything over 10 lbs for 6 weeks. (Ken)*

Long-term outcomes after adrenalectomy are not well described in the medical literature but here are some selected paragraphs from Carole A. Langrall (http://hyperaldosteronism.blogspot.com) who writes a blog about her experience with PA and adrenalectomy:

I noticed some effects immediately after surgery. As exhausted as I was in ICU- I still noticed the "brain fog" was gone, and this made me ecstatic. While I was on some heavy-duty drugs, I felt I was clear in my thinking and actions, and pretty alert considering I just had major surgery. My blood pressure was all over the place until 2 days later when it dropped lower that it had been in seven years. I was released from the hospital at that point.

Other changes were gradual, for example the polyuria was gone practically immediately. I started having quick bursts of energy within two weeks and got out of the house for a day trip. I fatigued easily though, so I would suggest limiting your physical activities for at least three weeks. As far as steps, do so but slowly. Don't think you will jump back into normal for at least a month.

I felt stronger within a month when I gradually resumed my work out routine at the gym. I no longer felt "confused" or whacked out, a side effect I suffered with a lot for the past two years. I also noticed the migraines had disappeared, as did the dehydration and muscle spasms at night.

Eight months later, there are some concerns that I plan to discuss with my doctor. Mainly- there is still some fatigue. As well, I have a difficult time with coffee (this stinks because I love it so...); I don't process sugar well, I crash immediately on it just as I do with wine or alcohol. My other adrenal seems to still be in recalibration mode, but certain stimulants do not take well.

In all, the major symptoms never came back--the high blood pressure is gone, as is the lowered potassium. The flank pain or kidney pain is also gone as is the dehydration, migraines, confusion (brain fog) and paresthesia. I have more energy than I can remember in a long time and forget this sometimes when I go all day without taking a break. Just typing those words makes me smile

Medications

Some good news is that there are some highly effective medications for PA. Multiple studies show that systolic blood pressure drops by an average of 20-32 mm and diastolic blood pressure an average of 9-12 mm in those with PA as a result of these drugs. This is a tremendous improvement for most patients. Studies using spironolactone to treat heart failure demonstrated a 30% reduction in mortality (death) compared to other treatments. Although a large multi-center trial of mediation use on cardiovascular outcomes in PA patients has not been performed, studies suggest that the drop in blood pressure noted from treatment will reduce the likelihood of fatal or nonfatal cardiovascular events.

In my case, starting on one of these drugs was a "miracle cure" that brought my elevated and volatile blood pressure to normal within days and kept it there relatively consistently. Not everyone will have that experience and there are potential side effects I have described for each medication (see below).

The bad news is that many people don't take their medications. A study of over 200 hypertensive patients found that 25% were completely or partially noncompliant with their medication prescription (10% not at all adherent) [71]. Researchers confirmed this by measuring the metabolites for the drugs in the urine of the individuals prescribed drugs. Although there are multiple reasons that people don't take prescribed drugs, including cost or side effects, many people simply forget to take them. I have some suggestions in the following section to help you remember to take your medications. However, if you believe this will be hard for you, you might pursue additional testing to determine whether surgery is an option.

Mineralocorticoid receptor blockers/antagonists

Spironolactone (brand name, Aldactone.

This is the first medication that was observed to cause substantial improvement of blood pressure in those with PA. This medication, used for other clinical conditions such as heart failure since the 1960s, binds to the same receptor as aldosterone and reduces the effects of aldosterone—it is an "antagonist" in that it has the opposite action as aldosterone. Some additional detail about this drug is provided below.

Doses and Pharmacology

Usually a patient is started on a low dose such as 12.5 mg and this is increased to as high as 200 mg per day in step-wise fashion, depending on the response. In other words, if your blood pressure normalizes when you are on 50 mg per day, this will likely be your prescribed dose unless something changes in the future.

The drug has a long half-life which means that it stays in the blood stream for a long time. Specifically, it takes about 14-16 hours for half of the dose to be fully eliminated by the body. This justifies the one dose per day regimen used for most people.

Mechanism of Action

Spironolactone reduces the opportunity for aldosterone to have effects throughout the body. Thus, even though aldosterone concentration in the blood remains high, it does not have the negative effects.

Remember that PA causes too much blood volume and sodium but abnormally low blood potassium. Spironolactone acts as a diuretic to increase loss of water and sodium from the blood which will produce more urine. Thus you may notice the need to urinate more during the day after you take it (possibly less at night if you experienced this symptom from untreated PA). Spironolactone causes the kidney to reduce retention of sodium while it increases potassium reabsorption. Since some of the negative symptoms of PA are caused by low blood potassium, this retention of potassium is valuable.

Side Effects

Spironolactone can be highly effective for PA, but it causes intolerable side effects in a subset of those taking it. Most of the side effects of spironolactone are related to its ability to also block the receptor for other hormones such as testosterone. This reduction in testosterone action is the reason that this drug is sometimes prescribed for acne. Up to 20% of men who take this drug develop "male boobs" (technically called gynocomastia) with erectile dysfunction (you know that term from all the commercials on television) and reduced libido (interest in sex). Women can experience menstrual disturbances and excess hair growth on atypical parts of the body (called hirsutism). Spironolactone can also be a mimic of prolactin, which can cause painful breasts in men or women.

The majority of people who take spironolactone do not have these side effects, but as you can imagine, those who experience them state they are intolerable and exclude this drug as a treatment choice. Talk to your doctor if you experience any of these effects. It is possible that a drop in dose may alleviate them. Or, you can try another medication.

An additional potentially serious side effect of using spironolactone is hyperkalemia, excessively high blood potassium. The specific definition of hyperkalemia may depend on the laboratory doing the measurement, but generally blood potassium greater than about 5.5 mmol/l could be of concern, while values above 6 mmol/l could be life threatening (Table 7). This side effect is more likely if you have kidney damage or are older. Hyperkalemia can be life threatening since it can result in heart arrhythmias (abnormal beating of the heart). Co-use of other drugs can also increase the risk of hyperkalemia, including some non-steroidal anti-inflammatory drugs (*e.g.*, naproxen, ibuprofen), ACE inhibitors, ARB (Table 11.). Still, high blood potassium as a result of spironolactone is relatively rare; the incidence is about 2-12% of patients taking spironolactone.

Interfering Substances

Specific drugs such as aspirin or NSAIDs such as naproxen or ibuprofen may reduce the effectiveness of spironolactone. Check with your doctor before taking these medications for pain or fever relief.

Continued Monitoring

Because of the risk of hyperkalemia, most doctors will measure your blood potassium after several weeks on spironolactone and at sporadic periods thereafter to insure normal blood potassium.

Patient Comments about Spironolactone

Some individuals report rapid improvement on spironolactone without any side effects. Those with side effects have generally reported that their doctors changed them to eplerenone.

> *Being female, I've never had a problem with spiro. My endo wanted me to try Inspra for some reason, he said it was new and more effective. I tried it for 3 weeks, 50 mg twice per day, the headaches got no better and my blood pressure was waaay high. Spiro seems to work well for me so I'll stick with it. (Shahall)*

> *saw a huuuge difference in my BP within 24 hours of starting spiro. I didn't get the full effect for a couple of weeks though. (Shahall)*

> *I ended up with Gynecomastia and Micropenis and it is not reversible after 12 months. (John)*

Eplerenone (brand name Inspra)

A newer drug that has most of the benefits for PA with fewer side effects was approved by the FDA in 2002 for essential hypertension and later for heart failure. Interestingly, it has not been officially approved for use in PA, mostly because the definitive studies showing improved mortality outcomes have not been done (and may never be done as they are very expensive). The challenge to this situation is that some patients with PA diagnosis may not have their eplerenone prescription covered by insurance, while they would if the official diagnosis was primary hypertension. Since it can be a highly effective treatment, work with your doctor to find a solution if eplerenone appears to be the best medication for you.

Originally, this drug was very expensive as you could not get it generically. The FDA rule is that a drug company that spends the substantial funds to develop a drug has a patent for 20 years with role as the only seller for about half of that time. Thus, since Pfizer developed the drug, it was the only company that could sell eplerenone (as the trade name Inspra) until 2011 with the final patents expiring in 2020 [56]. Now that other companies can produce it, the price has fallen substantially. Thus generic eplerenone has been available for prescription in the US for several years at the time of writing of this book. Apparently, it is not approved for use or available in some other countries.

Dose & Pharmacology

Eplerenone is about half as potent as spironolactone so the doses are typically higher. Typically, doctors will begin patients on a low dose, such as 25-50 mg per day, and raise this over a few weeks until reaching the appropriate blood pressure. Like spironolactone, there could be serious side effects if the dose is too high so it makes sense to use the lowest efficacious dose for you. The maximum approved dose is 100 mg per day although some doctors may prescribe higher doses if they believe this is the best treatment for the patient. Food does not affect absorption of the drug [56] so it does not matter if you take this drug on an empty stomach or with a meal.

Eplerenone is metabolized more quickly than spironolactone; it has a shorter half-life of approximately 3-4 hours (remember that this was 14-16 hours for spironolactone). For this reason, eplerenone is usually prescribed twice per day. Since patient compliance to medications goes down the more times per day medicines is prescribed, some doctors prescribe it only once per day. The peak blood concentration is expected about 1.5 hours after ingestion. Personally, my doctor prescribed a once per day dose. I moved the timing from morning to take the pill mid-day so that I would have maximum effect when I am likely to have higher stimulation of aldosterone because of sodium intake or physical activity (see later chapters). I checked with my doctor before I made this change. I also have no proof that this is a superior strategy for me, but it seemed to make sense based on the pharmacology of the drugs and my eating habits.

Many people see a rapid improvement within days of starting this medication. A steady state (consistent concentration in the blood) is usually achieved within two days.

Mechanism of Action

Eplerenone attaches to the mineralocorticoid receptor that normally binds aldosterone. Similar to spironolactone, it prevents aldosterone from having effects on the cell and stimulates opposite effects. Thus, the kidney will not retain excessive sodium and water allowing blood pressure to fall. Blood potassium typically rises since it causes potassium retention in the kidney.

Side Effects

A major value of eplerenone over spironolactone is that the former is less likely to bind with testosterone or progesterone receptors. Thus many of the side effects of spironolactone are not expected with this newer drug. Some people taking eplerenone will experience dizziness, headache, fatigue, diarrhea, an increase in blood urea nitrogen (BUN), high blood triglycerides, or high liver enzymes. These are not necessarily dangerous; your doctor can help you interpret any blood values that are outside the normal range. The side effects have a low occurrence but check with your doctor if you experience any unusual symptoms after you begin the drug.

Like spironolactone, eplerenone increases blood potassium. For many people with PA, this is a modest amount and is a welcome change since low blood potassium is associated with some of the symptoms of PA. However, very high blood potassium, above 5.5 mmol/L, is of concern and can be dangerous. If your blood potassium rises close to this level, this drug might be discontinued or reduced. The chance of this happening is unlikely but should be checked. A clinical trial using eplerenone in over 2700 heart failure patients showed that 4.6% more of the patients receiving eplerenone developed hyperkalemia than those on placebo [75]. In another trial, one of 68 patients on eplerenone while seven of 69 patients on spironolactone for 16 weeks developed hyperkalemia [59]. The risk of hyperkalemia is higher if you have kidney disease or if you are taking very high doses of the drug.

Interfering Substances

Eplerenone is metabolized in the liver by an enzyme called CYP3Af. So consumption of other drugs (or foods such as grapefruit) that also use this enzyme may interfere with the action of eplerenone. Examples include:

acetaminophen, codeine, erythromyocin, and diazepam. Check with your doctor or pharmacist to make sure any prescribed or over-the-counter drugs are appropriate when you are taking eplerenone.

Continued Monitoring

Similar to the procedure with spironolactone, your doctor is likely to ask you to come in for a blood sample within 10-14 days of starting eplerenone to check your blood potassium response. Sporadic subsequent check for blood potassium is usually recommended. If you notice any symptom of high blood potassium, including abnormally slow heart rate, erratic contraction, or unusual weakness contact your doctor.

Patient Comments about Eplerenone

Eplerenone has proved to work extremely well for me. My BP is controlled, I go to work daily, I coach two sports, and I participate in competitive sports. All of this at 37 years old. I am not trying to brag and I still have my challenging health days when I just don't feel right. However, I am able to catch up on fun things that I simply couldn't do before diagnosis and treatment 5 years ago. I generally eat between 2000 and 3500mg of sodium. This range seems to work well for me and still means I have to watch what I eat. (Scott)

I tried spirono[lactone] for over a year and had many problems with side effects. I have been on Eplerenone since August and have no side effects. I started at 50 mg, increased to 75 mg in November and with bp at 148/68 I will probably be increased to 100 mg when I see the doc on the 19th. (abrahmsp)

My nephrologist switched me from Spironolactone to Eplerenone but didn't double the dosage of Eplerenone (to what Spiro dosage is) so I ended up in the ER with critically low potassium. It was just an oversight but could have cost me my life, not to mention the inconvenience and expense of the ER. (Susie)

Spironolactone vs Eplerenone

From reading the information above, you can see some contrasts between these drugs in doses required, longevity of effect, incidence of side effects, and possibly price and availability. Remember that taking either spironolactone or eplerenone does not reduce the amount of aldosterone in your blood (and may actually increase it). It is, instead, interfering with the ability of aldosterone to attach to the receptor that stimulates many of the cellular changes you are trying to avoid.

Do studies show that one drug is more effective than the other for blood pressure reduction in PA patients? I found only a few studies that compared these two drugs directly in the same study. One [45] compared spironolactone in doses from 50-400 mg per day to eplerenone of 50-200 mg per day over 24 weeks in 37 PA patients. Both drugs were equally effective in reducing blood pressure. Another study [59] reported better reductions in blood pressure in patients taking spironolactone compared to those taking eplerenone. However, more male patients taking spironolactone developed female-like breasts and more female patients developed painful breasts. Overall, it appears that eplerenone is slightly less effective but better tolerated by most patients. The effects will be different by individual and there is no way to predict your reaction to the medications.

New Drug Development for Aldosteronism

Pharmaceutical companies are working on newer drugs, still in the experimental stage, that might be useful for PA. At least one compound that inhibits the synthesis of aldosterone -- currently named LC1699 -- has been tested in hypertensive patients [15]. A study of 14 PA patients with receiving LC1699 for four weeks reported that the drug caused a modest reduction in blood pressure, corrected low blood potassium, and caused a 75% reduction in blood aldosterone concentration. However, the reductions in blood pressure noted were significantly less than when these individuals were given eplerenone [3]. In addition, since the drug also partially inhibits the synthesis of cortisol, there is concern that this could impair the ability to react to stress [15]. More studies using longer testing periods with varied doses are required to evaluate whether this drug is safe or effective and if it has any benefit over currently available drugs.

Other Blood Pressure Medications

Less detail will be provided about these other medications since they are less specific to PA. Some common side effects will be provided but realize that these are not experienced by most people and that all drugs have potential side effects.

At least half of PA patients will need to take one or more of these drugs to normalize their blood pressure [50]. Why? Some patients may have other conditions that influence blood pressure such as obesity or atherosclerosis. These medications may be needed to act on different points of the regulation of blood pressure. Of course, there is a high prevalence of primary hypertension in the general population, so some patients with PA may have concurrent primary hypertension.

One study of PA patients 12 months after initiation of treatment with spironolactone [39] reported that most of the patients remained on other hypertensive drugs. About 88% continued to take a calcium channel blocker, 75% a diuretic, 63% either an ARB or ACEi, and 31% a beta-blocker. Interestingly, most patients who had an adrenalectomy were also still taking additional medicine for blood pressure (60% ACEi or ARB, 33% diuretic, 47% calcium channel blocker, 13% beta blocker).

It is possible that you might be able to go to mono-therapy, using only eplerenone or spironolactone. Work with your doctor to determine whether this is appropriate for you. A caution if you and your doctor decide to attempt to drop any medication—it is usually best to cut the dose in half, sequentially, for about a week rather than going "cold turkey" as some drugs cause tolerance that requiring weaning over time. This is especially true for some types of diuretics and beta- adrenergic blockers.

Table 11. Common Blood Pressure Medicines with their General Mechanism of Action

Medication Class	Example Generic Name	General Action
Thiazide-like diuretics	Chlorothiazide Hydrocholorothiazide Indapamide Chlorthalidone	Inhibit reabsorption of sodium (increase excretion sodium, potassium, and water) and in the distal tubule of the kidney; reduce blood volume
Loop diuretics	Bumetanide Furosemide	Reduce sodium reabsorption (increase excretion sodium, potassium, and water) at the loop of Henle in kidney; reduce blood volume
Potassium-sparing diuretics	Amiloride Triamterine	Inhibit the sodium channels in the distal convoluted tubule of the kidney; increase sodium and water excretion without potassium loss; reduce blood volume
Mineralocorticoid receptor blockers	Spironolactone Eplerenone	Antagonize the mineralocorticoid receptor to reduce effects of aldosterone on various cells in the body, including increased excretion of sodium and water by collecting duct cells of the kidney and relaxation of blood vessels
Beta-adrenergic blockers	Atenolol Bisoprolol Metoprolol Propanolol	Block the beta receptors for catecholamine hormones (*e.g.*, epinephrine) on receptors; reduce heart rate and relax muscles around blood vessels

Angiotensin converting enzyme inhibitor, ACEi	Captopril Enalapril Lisinopril	Inhibit the formation of angiotensin II from angiotensin I, reduce vasoconstriction and reduce production of aldosterone
Angiotensin receptor blocker, ARB	Candesartan Losartan Olmesartan Valsartan	Block the receptors that bind angiotensin II, reduce vasoconstriction and reduce production of aldosterone
Calcium channel blockers	Amlodipine Verapamil	Bind to calcium channels in heart and muscle cells; reduction in intracellular calcium can result in vasodilation and slower heart rate
Alpha + beta-blockers	Carvedilol Labetalol	Block both beta and alpha receptors for catecholamines in blood vessels, heart and brain; reduce heart rate and relax muscles around blood vessels

Note that this is not a complete list and you can check drug websites for information on the specific medications you take.

Diuretics

Diuretics act on the kidney to increase urine production and loss of body fluid. This helps to reduce excessive blood volume that may have caused elevated blood pressure. Some diuretics increase excretion of sodium, while others increase excretion of potassium along with the fluid loss. HCTZ (hydrochlorothiazide) is a common diuretic that is sometimes included with another drug in one pill (e.g. Losartan with HCTZ). HCTZ increases loss of potassium and so may not be tolerated by PA patients with low blood potassium.

A diuretic that is considered a "potassium sparing diuretic" is amiloride. This drug acts directly on the kidney to preferentially increase sodium excretion while retaining more potassium. Since excessive sodium retention and low blood potassium is a problem for PA, this is a drug your doctor may consider.

One potential concern about using diuretics is that they can indirectly increase production of aldosterone because of a reduction in kidney flow that occurs due to blood volume loss. This can be detected by the kidney, resulting in the production of renin to bring blood volume back up. As shown in Figure 3 this can stimulate an increase in angiotensin II and thus aldosterone—not a good thing for PA. For this reason, an angiotensin II reducing drug (see below) may be included with a diuretic.

Angiotensin-II interference

Angiotensin II is a potent vasoconstrictor that can contribute to high blood pressure. For many people with PA, angiotensin II will not be high since renin is suppressed. (Remember that renin helps convert angiotensin I to the active angiotensin II; see Figure 3.) However, it is possible that renin will be stimulated because of blood volume reduction from diuretics (see above) allowing an increase in angiotensin-II.

Reduction in the effects of angiotensin II can be accomplished by reducing its production via inhibition of the enzyme that is required to activate angiotensin. These drugs are called angiotensin converting enzyme inhibitors (ACEi) and include generic names like captopril and lisinopril.

Alternatively, the effects of angiotensin II can be reduced by blocking the receptor for this compound on the surface of cells. Angiotensin-II receptor blockers (ARB) include generic names like losartan and olmesartan. Usually, either an ACEi or an ARB, but not both, will be prescribed if a doctor believes suppression of angiotensin II is required to control your blood pressure.

ACE inhibitors sometimes cause a dry, annoying cough. An ARB is less likely to cause the cough. NSAIDs, antacids, and lithium may interfere with the action of ACE inhibitors

Beta- or alpha-adrenergic blockers

These drugs act on the muscle around blood vessels to encourage them to relax to open the vessels wider to reduce blood pressure. If the doctor believes part of your blood pressure problem might be related to over-contraction of the vessels, you might be prescribed a beta- or alpha-adrenergic blocker. I was prescribed carvedilol, a combination alpha- and beta- adrenergic blockers, but I apparently did not need it as eliminating it, after starting eplerenone, had no effect on my blood pressure.

Beta- or alpha-adrenergic blockers can cause fatigue and reduced exercise tolerance in some people. Heart rate is usually lowered and blood lipids may increase.

Remember—never decide on your own to stop or modify doses of drugs. Always check with your doctor and follow his/her advice on the best way to try eliminating a drug. Beta- or alpha-adrenergic blockers and diuretics are notoriously more difficult to stop than some other drugs. Usually, it is recommended to sequentially cut the dose over time before discontinuing. This time allows your body to adapt gradually.

Calcium channel blockers

These drugs reduce entrance of calcium into cells in the heart and blood vessels. This relaxes and widens the blood vessels and sometimes slows heart rate.

These drugs may have some of the common side effects of all blood pressure drugs such as fatigue, nausea, headache, but they also can cause heart arrhythmias in some people.

Drugs that may worsen hypertension

Drugs prescribed for another reasons can boost blood pressure. For example, oral contraceptive pills and some medications for arthritis can increase blood pressure. Some over-the-counter medications can increase blood pressure, including aspirin, non-steroidal anti-inflammatories (*e.g.*, naproxen, ibuprofen), cortisone, some antidepressants, and decongestants. If you are taking a diuretic and an ARB or ACEi, you should especially avoid aspirin or non-steroidal anti-inflammatory drugs. Since these drugs reduce the kidney blood flow, they can compromise kidney function and cause a rise in blood pressure through an increase in renin (termed "triple whammy") [17]. Some anti-depressant drugs (*e.g.*, Bupropion) or hyperactivity disorder drugs (*e.g.*, Ritalin) may increase your blood pressure. Finally, illicit drugs like cocaine, anabolic steroids, ecstasy, PCP, and amphetamine drugs acutely increase blood pressure. When I have a cold, I take over-the-counter medications designed for people with high blood pressure. Check with your pharmacist and on-line for side effects at sites like www.drugs.com/ for potential interactions of drugs you may be taking.

Surgery vs Medication Treatment

Surgery is only an option if you have excessive aldosterone from one adrenal, not if both of your adrenals are secreting excessive aldosterone. So if it is determined that you are eligible for surgery, should you do it? There are multiple things you might want to consider, including the severity of your PA, how well medications work for you, and your willingness to consistently take medication and control dietary sodium intake. You might also want to know whether one of these treatments shows evidence of better long- term health outcome.

Several studies have followed patients that chose surgery or medication treatment. Most studies show very similar improvements in blood pressure, resolution of cardiac abnormalities such as left ventricular hypertrophy, and reduction in kidney problems whether they did surgery or continued with medications. The improvements are usually observed more quickly with surgery, but in that case, you have to accept the potential complications from surgery.

One paper reported on 21 research studies that compared surgical to medical treatment of PA; six studies observed similar improvement of blood pressure and potassium, while the same number reported better improvement or fewer medications required following surgery [57]. The incidence of coronary heart disease, stroke, and heart arrhythmias were not different in patients who had been treated with medicine compared to surgery. The three studies that examined heart size showed that surgery and medicine were equally effective in reducing left ventricular mass, although the improvement happened more quickly in surgical patients. Three other studies that measured quality of life and psychological symptoms reported better outcome for surgical than medical treatment. Comparison among these studies is somewhat difficult since they were done in different clinics and varying follow-up periods.

Although I am willing to be diligent in taking multiple daily medications, many people are not. In a recent study of 1000 adults in the US, individuals were asked about their willingness to take a daily pill to reduce their risk of cardiovascular disease [38]. The researchers asked them how much of their life they would be willing to give up to avoid taking a daily, free medication. Although 70% said they were not willing to give up any life (*e.g.*, would take the pill), the remaining 300 people were willing to give up between one and 104 weeks of life to avoid taking a daily pill. Only you can decide whether or not you are willing to take your medications each day, likely for the rest of your life. It is an inconvenience I am willing to make. I am very appreciative that I have access to effective medications for PA.

Experimental Treatments

If you are not getting relief with traditional treatments, you might want to pursue experimental treatment. Researchers doing studies on PA will likely recruit subjects on sites like http://clinicaltrials.gov/ Go to this site and insert aldosterone or aldosteronism to see what trials may be going on. The site will typically describe the criteria for involvement, the purpose and procedures of the study, and provide contact information for someone who can answer your questions. You can typically apply to be considered for the trial on-line. They will contact you if you qualify.

One attraction of this approach is that the studies typically pay for any medical or surgical procedures they do. Some patients have been accepted for evaluation at an NIH lab in Maryland that covers everything from AVS to surgery. They offer this in order to learn more about the disease as well as to train physicians on the procedures. The obvious downsides are that you will not be able to select the treatment you receive if they are testing several approaches. In addition, you will have to travel to their site in Maryland and possibly stay there for a prolonged period or return several times at your own expense.

You can find Internet posts from individuals who have been through the NIH testing lab such as this below:

> *Got awakened at 5:30 as promised and my nurse tried to get an IV line in my right arm.... So, then the fun began. First, go pee, for the 24 hour, and then another for the test coming up, plain urinalysis. Then, they started the saline suppression test... So, after the saline suppression test (4- -5 hours of sitting still with my arms not moving so as to not make the alarms go off on the saline and keep the other line open), I was taken to Radiology for the CT with contrast.... it was done fairly quickly. Then I was wheeled back upstairs, given water, thank god, and after a bit more of a blood draw, was seen again by another cardiologist.... I met Dr. ---- and spoke with him at length. I now know everything there is to know about PA and all these tests. Furthermore, he answered every question I asked, and pulled up my "normal" MRI from a couple months ago, and showed me the abnormal left adrenal gland..... it was a rough day to get through physically, but I am still very grateful to be here and feel very well cared for. (Maggie)*

Patients are typically required to withdrawal from many blood pressure medications for 4-6 weeks before the NIH testing and use substitute drugs like verapamil and hydralazine that are less likely to influence the results of tests. This means you should be prepared to work with them for months. One patient described the multiple tests she went through during one NIH lab visit: five days in a row of 24 h urine collection, several blood collections, echocardiogram, and the AVS procedure.

Is Remission Possible?

Although rare, there have been reports in the medical literature about remission in patients with PA. For example, one Japanese man had refused surgery for his adrenal tumor observed on a CT scan but took spironolactone for five years [74]. After the five years, a repeat of diagnostic tests showed no evidence of PA and dramatic improvement of his left ventricular hypertrophy. Another case study describes a 41-year-old patient with APA who also did not want to undergo surgery and was treated with spironolactone for 15 years. When he decided to undergo surgery instead of continuing on the medication, his aldosterone measured normal and PA was not deemed to be present.

The German Conn registry collects data on PA patients. A report from this group calculated a remission rate of approximately 5.4% in the patients they studied [22]. An Italian research group did ARR and a saline infusion test on 34 patients who had been diagnosed between three and 15 years earlier (47). All had been receiving medication treatment since diagnosis. Seventy-six percent of these patients were not confirmed to have PA in this follow-up test. They found that female gender and higher blood potassium during treatment were associated with a higher chance that PA was resolved. This particularly high proportion of resolved PA is promising but should be confirmed in additional studies.

So although rare, remission is possible. There is not enough information at this time, to predict who may have a remission or if you can do anything in particular to encourage remission.

Chapter 8

LIVING WELL WITH PA

If you've chosen medication as a means to control your PA, this section may help you make the best decisions on managing your condition. Don't give up your health as the sole responsibility of your physician. Take control of your own health by paying attention to your body, keeping accurate records of symptoms and medical tests, eating a diet that may help you control PA, and continuing to learn about the latest information and new developments.

Pay Attention to your Body

Everyone has unique reactions to this condition and to the medications. Paying attention to symptoms may help your doctor accurately treat your condition. He/she will want specifics. Things like "I felt dizzy" are not as useful as "I felt dizzy first thing in the morning, starting three days after I began the new diuretic medication". Although you think you will remember it all, I found it useful to keep a small notebook to record the existence and timing of various symptoms as well as my blood pressure. For example, I recorded when I felt chest "pinching" or when I had a whooshing sound in my ears. I added anything unusual as far as my diet or physical activity. Can you see any patterns? For example, do you notice more trouble after you eat at a restaurant? After hard exercise? After a stressful day? After you've taken a supplement or over-the-counter drug? These are all valuable observations that could be useful information to your doctor.

Taking Accurate Blood Pressure Measurements

Not long ago, patients had to go into their doctor's office any time they wanted to know their blood pressure. Today there are relatively inexpensive home monitors that open up the ability to measure blood pressure easily, regularly, and accurately. These home monitors are also useful for people who get "white coat hypertension," an increase in blood pressure due to the stress of being at a doctor's office.

The value of home blood pressure monitors on clinical outcome was demonstrated in a 1-year study comparing high-risk hypertensive patients checking their blood pressure at home with permission to modestly modify medications depending on readings, compared to a group who sporadically came into the doctor's office for measurement and advice on medication [51]. At the end of the study, the home monitoring patients had a 9.2 mm greater blood pressure reduction than those relying on the doctor's measurements and management.

Ask your doctor for a recommendation on brand of blood pressure monitor. Arm cuff monitors are typically more accurate than finger or wrist monitors and are easy to use. You can buy these monitors in drug stores, superstores, or on-line. Expect to pay $40-100. My doctor recommended the Omron brand. There are different size cuffs depending on your arm size (measure it with a tape measure and check against recommendations on box). If you have very large upper arm circumference, you may need the larger size. Using a too small a cuff will result in an incorrectly high blood pressure. If the cuff is too large, it may not provide a reading at all or be incorrectly low for you.

Your insurance company may pay for the monitor or provide a discount. Ideally, you should test the accuracy of the monitor you get by bringing it with you on your next doctor visit. Take your blood pressure using the monitor a few minutes after they have taken it at the office. Look for a reading within about 5 mm.

At home, take your blood pressure when seated quietly for about five minutes. Keep both feet on the floor and do not cross your legs. Since caffeine or nicotine can modestly increase blood pressure and heart rate, avoid having caffeine or smoking within 30 minutes of your blood pressure measurement. Make sure the cuff is placed appropriately. This means placing it on bare upper arm with the mark on cuff lined up with center of inside of your elbow (at the brachial artery). The bottom of the cuff should be about an inch above the elbow crease. (Read the instructions). Take the pressure while sitting quietly and not talking. It is best to take 2-3 readings each time and average the last two. Keep a record of the pressures with any notation about factors that could have influenced it (*e.g.,* forgot to take medicine yesterday, ate a high sodium meal). This record will be useful in locating patterns and predictors of your blood pressure. Bring it with you to the doctor to show the level of control you are achieving.

Blood pressure typically varies throughout the day, so you may want to get some readings at different times. Morning blood pressure is often the highest since your nervous system revs up to help you wake up. Mine is usually higher later in the day. Once you get a sense of the change in your blood pressure over the day, select one time to consistently take it so you can compare day to day.

Physical activity increases blood pressure, so avoid taking it within 30-45 minutes of an exercise session. Blood pressure drops for most people about 15-25% at night. Lack of a blood pressure drop at night, termed "nondippers," is actually a sign of cardiovascular risk.

Keep Accurate Records

When I knew I had high blood pressure but had no idea what was causing it, I keep meticulous, careful records of my blood pressure each day. I was looking for triggers that I could associate with the unexplained swings to high pressures I experienced. During this period, one doctor asked how often I was taking my blood pressure. When I said daily (and sometimes multiple times during a day of variation), he said I should stop and maybe take it once a week. He thought anxiety about my blood pressure was pushing it higher. I argued that I did not believe anxiety would cause the very high systolic pressures I was seeing. My opinion is that, especially when you are trying to figure out the cause of your hypertension or when you alter your medications or diet, you do regular and consistent blood pressure measurement with a home monitor. Now that I am more reliably in control, I only take my blood pressure every two weeks or so unless I feel unusual symptoms.

Working with Your Medical Team

Look at yourself as part of the team managing your condition. Provide pertinent information that may be useful to the doctor, and have specific questions prepared ahead. Avoid too many questions that may irritate your busy physician but don't hesitate to ask for more explanation or ask why certain things are recommended. You (or your insurance company) are paying him/her for this treatment that should include educating and working with you. Avoid feeling guilty that you are taking up too much time. Although a doctor may have to put in some extra time to investigate treatment of PA, the knowledge and experience they gain will help them treat future patients.

Doctors are often forced to keep office visits short. So, be prepared ahead with your list of a handful of key questions. Take notes on their responses. Avoid asking too many trivial questions and focus on the most important ones that will influence your treatment.

Taking Medication Consistently

Although skipping your medication occasionally is unlikely to cause major problems, consistent use of medication is critical for the best control of your condition. That means take the same dose, at similar time of the day each day. Be sure to follow the instructions on taking them on an empty stomach or with food, as advised by the pharmacy. You can use different methods to make this easier for you to remember. Some people always take their medications in the morning with breakfast. You might buy one of the plastic boxes with compartments labeled for each day of the week. This helps you on those days where you wonder whether you already took your medicines. If you have been prescribed medicine more than once per day, you might again consistently pair it with a meal to remind you—*e.g.*, take the pill every day before dinner. I give myself two reminders for taking my eplerenone pill at noon. I set my cell phone alarm and use a free texting service that sends me a daily text message at noon to remind me to take my medication.

Ask your doctor or pharmacist what to do if you forget a pill. In other words, should you just wait until the next day or take it late that same day with resumption of normal schedule the following day? Taking medication correctly and consistently can help reduce symptoms as well as long-term complications of PA.

Diet for PA

Licorice

There is one unusual dietary practice that can cause symptoms similar to PA, excessive consumption of licorice! A chemical in licorice, glycyrrhizin, can mimic the symptoms of PA. Ceasing consumption of licorice cures the problem. I assume this is rare but have not seen any estimate of the number of cases caused by excessive licorice ingestion. If you don't eat excessive amounts of licorice, you can eliminate this as a cause of your hypertension and move onto other dietary management strategies.

Sodium

None of my doctors ever mentioned that I should restrict my dietary sodium. However, I read about the importance of dietary sodium on Internet PA forums and in scientific articles. Remember that blood sodium is a trigger to routinely increase the release of aldosterone. The normal body reaction after blood sodium attains an appropriate level is to reduce production of aldosterone, and thus stop retaining sodium. However, in aldosteronism, the adrenals ignore this shut-off signal so that excessive sodium intake can result in very high blood aldosterone concentration.

Technical Discussion #4

Sodium and Blood Pressure

There is evidence that the combination of high blood sodium with high aldosterone is particularly dangerous to tissues (Table 12). Early research on rats demonstrated that injection of aldosterone in rats caused heart fibrosis only when it was paired with a high sodium diet. Human trials studying the interaction of sodium consumption on complications from hypertension are limited and almost none focus on PA *per se*. Still, these few human studies show that combining a high sodium diet with high blood aldosterone is a problem. Note that since dietary sodium is not easy to quantify (diet records are usually not very accurate), most of these studies use the total amount of sodium lost in urine over one day as a surrogate for dietary sodium.

Table 12. Connection of Sodium with Aldosterone, Blood Pressure and Organ Damage

Example Evidence for a Connection between Sodium Intake and Hypertension:
a. Correlation between dietary/urinary sodium and blood pressure in over 10,000 men and women from 52 centers around the world [41].   b. Reduction in blood pressure (average approximately 3.7 mm systolic and 7 mm diastolic) when hypertensive patients reduce their dietary sodium [61].   c. A 25% reduction in risk of cardiovascular event when pre-hypertensive patients reduced dietary sodium [16].   d. A meta-analysis of 17 trials representing 734 hypertensive patients calculated that a modest reduction in salt intake for 4 weeks or more had an important effect on blood pressure that would predict reduction in stroke of 14% and coronary deaths by 9% [35].
Example Evidence of Connection of Sodium Intake to Organ Damage in Hypertensive Patients:
a. Correlation between urinary sodium and urinary protein (index of kidney damage) [23].   b. Improvement in left ventricular heart mass in treated hypertensive patients correlating to the change in urinary sodium and blood

aldosterone [19].

Example Evidence Connecting Sodium Plus High Aldosterone to Organ Damage:
a. Cardiac fibrosis occurred with administered aldosterone to rats *only* when simultaneous infusion of salt [9]. b. Urinary sodium correlated to heart thickening (left ventricular hypertrophy) in patients with PA [61]. c. Correlation between urinary protein excretion (index of kidney damage) and urinary sodium excretion *only* in those with high blood aldosterone [62]. d. Correlation of heart thickening (left ventricular hypertrophy) with urinary sodium and aldosterone excretion in 317 untreated PA patients [44].

Sodium Craving

Interestingly, aldosterone appears to have a role in appetite for sodium. In other words, elevated aldosterone tends to increase craving for salt. When the receptors for aldosterone in rats were blocked with spironolactone, sodium appetite was reduced [24]. So it is possible that you noticed that you desired more salty foods when PA was developing and that this was relieved when you got the correct medication or surgery.

End Technical Discussion #4

What is the Recommended Intake of Sodium?

The American Heart Association and the US Dietary Guidelines recommend that all American adults should consume no more than 2300 mg of sodium per day and that many individuals (all adults older than 50, all African American adults, and all adults with hypertension, diabetes, or kidney disease) should consume no more than 1500 mg per day (Table 13). How close are most people to this amount? Not close. The average sodium intake in the US is approximately 3400 mg per day. Less than 12% of the US population who should consume 2300 mg of sodium do so and less than 1% of those who should consume 1500 mg per day or less (according to the above guidelines) do.

Table 13. Dietary Sodium and Potassium Recommendations

Nutrient	Recommendation		Average Intake in US
	Adults	Over age 50 or African American or hypertensive	
Sodium	2300 mg per day	1500 mg per day	3400 mg per day
Potassium	4700 mg per day		2640 mg per day

The dietary sodium recommendations have been discussed recently in the medical literature and the news. Although most nutrition and medical scientists and societies agree that people should consume less than 2300 mg per day, the recommendation to move sodium intake lower to 1500 mg is more controversial [40]. A few studies find higher mortality at very low sodium take [58]. Critics of these studies suggest this is because people at the low end of sodium intake are either already sick and not eating much food or have such severe illness that they have been stringent about reducing their sodium intake [4].

Regardless of whether it is helpful or necessary to reduce sodium intake to 1500 mg per day, most agree that average sodium intake is too high and should be reduced to at most ~2300 mg per day. Some of the media have over-interpreted studies criticizing the very low sodium recommendation by saying that sodium no longer matters [4]. There is vast evidence that the typical high sodium intake (greater than 2300 mg) can be harmful to the health of many people (see Table 12).

Remember that all these recommendations for sodium were made for average Americans, not those with PA or even hypertension. We know sodium is a primary and powerful stimulator of aldosterone secretion. You will feel better, likely need less medication, and have less chance of organ damage if you follow a lower sodium diet. My opinion is that you should move as close to 1500 mg per day as possible. You may not reach that every day but it is a good target for your average intake. In order to achieve this sodium intake, you likely will need to severely limit the foods contributing most to sodium intake in the US. This means selecting low sodium versions of foods, avoid eating out, and prepare much of your own food. Tips on achieving your sodium goal will be covered later in this chapter.

PA patients have posted comments about improvement in how they feel when they eat a lower sodium diet. I personally feel bloated if I splurge on a higher sodium meal (usually if I eat out or attend a party). Eating a lower sodium diet may allow a lower dose of mineralocorticoid receptor blocker. See this comment from an Internet post:

I'm on 100mg of eplerenone/day..... I feel many could step down their MCB [mineralocorticoid receptor blocker] once they understand the requirement to keep Na [sodium] low and K [potassium] high. I think many doctors increase the dose without considering or even knowing that Na plays a major role. I know my PCP has never suggested eliminating or reducing the dose of any med. In fact I have to suggest it (or I do it myself). (John)

It can be confusing to estimate your total sodium as compared to salt (sodium chloride) intake. Salt contains chloride as well as sodium so you need to do some mathematical conversion to estimate sodium if you know the amount of salt or *visa versa*. Specifically, salt is 40% sodium. The magic number to remember for the conversion is 2.5. If you have the milligrams of salt in a food, divide this by 2.5 to get the milligrams of sodium. To convert sodium to salt, multiple by 2.5 (Table 14). Remember that there will always be less sodium by weight than salt in a food—this should help you remember whether you should multiply or divide by 2.5. If you need to go from milligrams to grams, you divide milligrams by 1000 (move the decimal three places) whereas going from grams to milligrams requires multiplication by 1000.

Table 14. Sample Conversions Sodium and Salt

10 g of salt divided by 2.5 = 4 g of sodium
1200 mg of sodium times 2.5 = 3000 mg of salt
1000 mg of sodium = 1 g of sodium

Not all the sodium we consume comes from sodium chloride (salt). Some may be as food additives such as sodium sulfite, sodium phosphate, sodium nitrite, or monosodium glutamate to name a few. The more processed foods you eat, the more chance you have of consuming sodium from these sources.

The Center for Science in the Public Interest (see: www.cspinet.org/salt/) states that sodium is "probably the single most harmful substance in the food supply." And "reducing sodium consumption by half would save an estimated 100,000 lives per year." The Center for Disease Control and Prevention calls dietary sodium "a critical public health issue." The World Health Organization, National Academy of Sciences, American Medical Association, and the US Department of Health and Human Services all agree that we should reduce our sodium intake. However, no regulations have been imposed to encourage companies or restaurants to change their food offerings or recipes. The sodium content of items at eight leading fast food chains actually rose more than 20% between 1997 and 2010 [13].

Where Is the Most Sodium in Our Foods?

It is astounding how much sodium is added to most processed and prepared foods. Go to the website of any chain restaurant or see the label on many foods. You will be shocked to see the sodium content of items on the menus and available at the grocery store. Most fast food burgers with condiments and toppings, for example, contain 1000-2000 mg alone, without the salted fries you might buy with them.

So what can you do if you want to try to reduce your sodium intake towards the recommended targets? The Center for Disease Control and Prevention [CDC] analyzed the US diet to determine which foods contributed the most to our sodium intake. The results might surprise you. Most of my students incorrectly guess "potato chips" or "pickles" as the highest sodium contributor to our diet. These are high sodium foods, but most of us don't eat enough of them to reach the top of this list. The food group contributing most to our sodium consumption is "breads and rolls." It isn't that one serving is so high—one slice of bread may have 150-250 mg of sodium—but that we eat so much of this food group in our daily diet. See Table 15 for the rank and contribution of the ten food groups to total sodium in the average American diet. Together, these food groups represent about 40% of the average total sodium intake.

You might be surprised to see "poultry" at number 4. Most uncooked or cooked poultry we buy has been injected or processed with added sodium. This is done to increase tenderness and/or weight since sodium increases water retention in the meat. The sodium also alters the taste and rate of spoilage. Your personal ranked list of top sodium contributors is likely not identical to this national average. However, it makes sense to start with this list to focus on reducing the amount of sodium you eat. Reduce the amount of foods within these groups or find lower sodium versions (discussed later).

TABLE 15 Table 15. Contribution of Food Groups to the Total US Sodium Intake [CDC]

Rank	Food Group	% Contribution to Total Sodium Intake
1	Breads & rolls	7.4%
2	Cold cuts/cured meats	5.1
3	Pizza	4.9
4	Poultry	4.5
5	Soup	4.3
6	Sandwiches	4.0
7	Cheese	3.8
8	Pasta mixed dishes	3.3
9	Meat mixed dishes	3.2
10	Savory snacks	3.1

Sodium- Safer foods

Some foods are so low in sodium that you can eat them, in normal quantities, without concern about their contribution to daily sodium intake. For example, the following foods purchased as the version without added flavoring or sauces and consumed without adding salt during cooking will not contribute substantially to your sodium intake:

Table 16. Sodium-Safer Foods

Air-popped popcorn
Beverages such as coffee, tea, seltzer water
Chocolate*+
Dried beans or no-salt-added canned beans
Eggs*
Fresh or frozen fruits and vegetables without sauce
Fresh or frozen beef* or fish (no sauces or flavoring added, avoid smoked, shellfish tend to be higher than other fish)
Jams, jellies, honey+
Oils or no salt butter*
Pasta, rice, or other grains (cooked without added salt)
Rolled oats, flour
Spices (e.g. cinnamon, basil, rosemary; NOT most spice blends like steak seasoning that often have salt as a primary ingredient)
Vinegar

* indicates high in fat, + indicates high in sugar

These are items you need not track of for purposes of sodium intake. If you are trying to lose weight, are diabetic, or have high blood lipids, control of the items that are high in fat or sugar should be considered. For PA, the primary dietary focus is on sodium.

On the other hand, Table 17 provides a list of foods that should not be consumed or should be consumed only sparingly if you are trying to eat a low sodium diet.

Table 17. Sodium-Caution Foods

Bacon or other cured or smoked meats
Olives
Pickles or other pickled foods
Salt and salty spice mixes
Sauerkraut
Soup or bouillon (regular)
Soy and other Asian sauces (regular)

Do not be confused that "sea salt" is any more healthful than regular salt. Also be careful that "lite" or lower fat foods often have higher sodium content. Check the label!

Calculating and Keeping Track of Sodium Intake

Most patients do not receive information about diet from their physicians. Registered dietitians can be an important component of your medical team. They are trained to help you achieve a low sodium diet. If your doctor has not recommended a dietitian, go to the Academy of Nutrition and Dietetics website (http://www.eatright.org/). Click on the "find a registered dietitian" button. You can search by your area code. A list will be provided with their address and email. You can refine your search to only those that have expertise in "heart health."

If you would prefer to work on a low sodium diet on your own, I recommend you begin keeping track of and becoming more aware of sodium in your diet. The old fashioned method is to write down everything you eat, look up the sodium content, and calculate intake total for the day. The American Heart Association has a free "sodium tracker" template you can download for this use (go to: www.heart.org and search for "sodium tracker"). Careful record keeping might be especially helpful as you get started modifying your diet. This process will help you highlight which foods in your diet contribute the most sodium. Overtime, you may decide you don't need to carefully quantify the sodium each day, but if you feel your diet is getting sloppy, start again.

The American Heart Association has a "Sodium Breakup" website (http://sodiumbreakup.heart.org/) with resources to help you reduce your sodium intake. You can sign up to receive the regular blog from "Suzie Sodium", find educational articles, read comments about related medical research, download an infographic, or watch videos about sodium. You can share your sodium story at the website for possible inclusion in the blog post.

Most books that list the nutritional content of food will include values for sodium. Realize these values are averages and that the particular brand or recipe you use may not be in the book's list. Pay attention to the serving size used for the book values. The package size is rarely the same as the serving size. If the listed serving size doesn't match what you actually ate, you'll need to do some math to estimate your sodium intake. For example, if the label says a serving is 3 oz. with 300 mg of sodium, you will need to double the sodium estimate if you eat 6 oz. of that food. Keep a list of all foods and drinks over the day with brand names and specific quantities to get a sense of your total sodium intake. After keeping careful records of what you eat for a week or two, you may learn to accurately estimate your sodium intake without writing it down.

Throughout this book, I have provided sodium content for various foods that I obtained from company websites, labels, or nutrition databases. Of course, recipes used by manufacturers or restaurants change over time. The sodium content I have provided could have changed by the time you read this book if companies changed formulations. These are used as examples rather than absolute fact. Be sure to check the label and updated websites!

If you are comfortable with technology, there are many Internet sites that can help you determine the sodium content of foods. The free USDA SuperTracker site can be located on Choose My Plate website. (http://www.choosemyplate.gov/). You can use the tool to quantify the nutrients you are eating, including sodium. You can look up the nutrient content for single foods or enter your entire day to get a sense of your sodium intake. You can even create a profile, save what you've entered, and keep track of your diet over time. You can create a "favorite foods" list that will make entering easier if you tend to eat similar foods day to day. Notice that you can also enter physical activities to get a sense of the number of calories you are expending each day. This is valuable if you are trying to lose weight. Although the SuperTracker tool may have a steeper learning curve than others, it likely has the best, largest database and most accurate values of those available for free.

Other diet analysis websites include "MyFitnessPal," "LoseIt," "CRON-O-Meter," and "Spark People," among others. The links to these sites are provided in Table 18. All of these sites have free versions while some have a pay version with more services. Some of them have a recipe analysis tool that may be useful if you are creating lower sodium recipes. Use the values you obtain from these sites as estimates rather than truth as many of the listings have not been verified. For example, I found a listing that said one raw potato had 10.6 g of sodium. This is outrageous and untrue—the true content is about 13 mg of sodium, over 800 times different. I trust the USDA site, My Plate and SuperTracker, the most.

Many of these sites are geared towards weight loss since that is frequently why people want to assess their diets. However, you can use them even if you are comfortable with your weight but want to focus on sodium intake. Most of the websites have "communities" that allow interaction among people with similar interests. I found several "communities" on the sites listed in Tale 18 that focused on eating lower sodium diets or cooking recipes lower in sodium.

Table 18. Example Free On-line Diet Analysis Sites

Name	Web address
Lose it	www.loseit.com
My Fitness Pal	www.myfitnesspal.com
Spark People	www.sparkpeople.com
USDA SuperTracker	www.choosemyplate.gov

Since the majority of people in the US now have smart phones (58% in 2014 according to the Pew Research Internet Project), mobile apps have been created to assess your complete diet or only your sodium intake. Many of the websites listed in Table 18 have a companion mobile application. Some apps are free and others have a modest up-front cost. Some are available only for certain types of phones (*e.g.*, Android, iPhone). Examples for complete diet analysis available at this time include: "Fooducate," "MyNetDiary." One valuable feature with some apps is data entry via barcode scanning of packaged foods. "Restaurant Nutrition" has nutritional information on 1000s of restaurant items. Other smart phone apps are specific to sodium such as "EZ Sodium Tracker." I do not advocate one of these websites or apps over another but point them out as ones you might try. Read the users comments to see concerns and opinions.

A critical issue with any of these tracking approaches is the quality of your data entry. Can you accurately estimate the portion size of what you eat? Most people cannot. Even people who are well trained in nutrition tend to underestimate portion sizes. One study comparing female dietitians to non-dietitians showed that the dietitians were more accurate than the non-dietitians but still underestimated their caloric intake by about 223 calories per day compared to the 429 calories underestimate by the non-dietitians. [12]

One way to improve your estimating ability is to literally weigh or measure the volume of what you are eating with a scale or measuring cups for a few days. You can also use props to estimate portion sizes. For example, a half-cup of cooked rice or pasta is about the size of a tennis ball. A medium baked potato listed in food analysis tables would be comparable to the size of a computer mouse. One-fourth cup of raisins is about the size of an egg. Two tablespoons of peanut butter is about the size of a Ping-Pong ball. Finally, 3 oz. of cooked meat, fish, or poultry is about the size of a deck of cards or the palm of your hand. You can find various websites with tips on estimating portion size (e.g., http://www.webmd.com/diet/healthtool-portion-size-plate).

American's average portion size is creeping higher. According to an National Institutes of Health website, the size of an average bagel was three inches 20 years ago but is six inches today. Even more dramatic, an average blueberry muffin 20 years ago was about 1.5 oz. but today is more than three times that at 5 oz. Accurately entering the portion size is essential in obtaining accurate nutrient reports.

I tend to have a few "go to" meals that I know are lower in sodium and nutritious. Then I do not need to repeatedly record and calculate the sodium content. See Table 19 for some examples of meals I eat that are lower in sodium.

Table 19. Examples of Lower Sodium Meals and Snacks

Breakfast	mg sodium*
Oatmeal or shredded wheat cereal+ milk + ½ cup berries	0 + 122 + 0 (122)
2 poached eggs + 1 slice lower sodium toast + fruit	147 + 140 + 1 (288)
1 cup plain low-fat yogurt + 1 apple + ¼ cup lower sodium granola	159 + 1 + 8 (168)
Lunch	
2 oz. lower sodium bread with lower sodium roast beef + lettuce/tomato + orange	280 + 40 + 2 (322)
Salad with 3 cups of mixed greens and vegetables + 3 oz. grilled chicken breast + 2 T lower sodium dressing	15 + 63 + 110 (188)
Dinner	
6 oz. baked salmon + roasted vegetables + 1	210 + 20 + 2 (232)

cup rice with homemade no-salt seasoning 5 oz. chicken kabob with low sodium plum sauce + 1 cup rice with homemade no-salt seasoning	195 + 2 (197)
Snacks	
Lightly salted roasted almonds, 1 oz. Low sodium rice cake with 1 T low sodium peanut butter	40 (40) 15 + 40 (55)

Sodium values show the addition of each item within the row with the total for the meal or snack in parenthesis.

Restaurants

It is very hard to eat a low sodium diet if you eat in restaurants or choose fast-food. One meal can easily hit or go beyond your sodium target for the day. A breakfast of a country ham and egg biscuit at Burger King will give you almost 1980 mg of sodium while a Hardee's Monster Thickburger clocks in at about 1200 mg (Table 20). You might think salads are harmless, but an Au bon Pain Greek salad with shrimp has approximately 1380 mg, with the dressing adding about 310 mg.

Table 20. Example "Sodium Busters" at Restaurants

Item	Sodium (mg)
Applebee's quesadilla burger	3260
Au Bon Pain turkey Cubano on ciabatta	2030
Burger King country ham and egg biscuit	1980
Hardees 2/3 pound monster Thickburger	2820
PF Chang's almond and cashew chicken	3780
Baja fresh carnitas with flour tortillas	3450
Olive Garden tour of Italy	3830

One piece of pizza can be 400-900 mg per slice depending on where you buy it and what you have on it (Table 21). An individual described his handling a lower sodium diet saying that if he knew he was having a high sodium dinner (like restaurant pizza), he would prepare for that by eating a very sodium- restricted diet earlier in the day.

Table 21. Sodium Content per Slice (mg) by Topping on Pizza

Mushroom and green pepper	Pepperoni	Bacon Cheeseburger
530	700	830

Domino's hand-tossed, 14 inch size used as an example, from their website. Check company websites for different brands.

I'm not picking on these restaurants as they are no different than most. I use these examples to illustrate that it's easy to bust your goal of 1500 mg per day or even 2300 mg per day sodium goal with just one meal eating out unless you choose lower sodium options. See Table 22 using Panera as an example menu with a wide variety of sodium content items. Remember that you can get the sodium content of most chain restaurant offerings on-line or ask on site.

I love to eat at restaurants but try to limit the number of times per week that I dine out. And I've learned to check the nutrition information, if available, before I go. Most restaurants will provide a list of the sodium content of their offerings on site or you can find this on-line. Since 2010, restaurants with at least 20 branches are required to provide nutritional information of their dishes to customers. In 2014, the FDA issued a requirement that restaurants as well as grocery stores and vending machines post the calorie information of their food items at the point of sale. Restaurants will have one year and vending machines two years to comply. Single establishments or smaller chains do not have to provide this information. Since they are only required to list calories, you may still have to ask or look on their website for sodium content.

I often try to plan for a restaurant meal by eating very low sodium during the day prior to the dinner out. I will look at an on-line menu, if available, before I go, to see what choices might be close to 1000 mg of sodium. (For examples, see Table 22). Believe me, there will not be many that are that low in sodium.

Table 22. Learn to Find the Lower Sodium Items on a Menu—Panera

Item	Amount	Sodium (mg)
Higher Sodium Choices		
French onion soup	1 cup	1460
Large macaroni and cheese	1 serving	2470
Sierra turkey sandwich on focaccia	1 sandwich	1930
Greek salad with shrimp + 3 T dressing	1 whole salad	1380 + 310
Tomato and mozzarella on ciabatta panini	1 sandwich	1550
Smoked ham and Swiss on rye	1 sandwich	2250
Pickle spear side	1	410
Baguette side	2.5 oz.	440
Lower Sodium Choices		
Creamy tomato soup	1 cup	340
Tuna salad on whole wheat	1 sandwich	1150
Mediterranean egg white on ciabatta	1 sandwich	830
Steel cut oatmeal with crunch topping, strawberries and pecans	1 serving	160
Roasted turkey & avocado BLT on sourdough	1 sandwich	980
Wild salmon Caesar salad + 3 T dressing	whole salad	640 + 210
Apple side	1	0
Potato chip side	1 package	170

Information from company website

Once you observe the sodium content of foods, you will be better able to select from menus that don't provide sodium content of each dish. For example, breading on chicken will boost sodium content, most commercial tomato sauces are high in sodium, and almost all Asian or Greek dishes are high in sodium because of the sauces and cheese/olives they contain. Does that mean you can never have your beloved stir-fry Thai food again? You have a few choices—make it yourself substituting lower sodium versions of ingredients, ask the chef at a restaurant to reduce the amount of the high sodium ingredients, or eat only a small portion. For example, you could share the Thai stir-fry with a friend and order a large helping of plain white rice so that you dilute the sodium content of the meal.

What will happen if you overdo your sodium intake one day? If you have a big event or holiday meal where you just didn't focus on sodium intake, you can overwhelm the medicine you are taking such that you have more aldosterone secreted than the medicine can block. You might notice some water retention (weight gain and bloated feeling) and possibly a rise in blood pressure. If this happens, make up for the slip the next day with a super low sodium day. Do not take any additional pills unless recommended by your doctor. For example, taking an extra diuretic may expel some of your excessive sodium that has been retained but may push your blood potassium too low.

Cooking Low Sodium

The best way to know what is in foods you are eating is to prepare them yourself. Learn to read ingredient food labels. Check out low- sodium recipes on-line or in cookbooks. The American Heart Association has a great low sodium recipe book. Buy reduced- sodium ingredients to use in recipes you already enjoy. I love Asian food but am cautious about eating this at restaurants as they often load it with high sodium sauces and MSG. I buy reduced-sodium Asian sauces at the grocery store or on-line (see www.lowsaltfoods.com or www.healthyheartmarket.com) so that I can make this cuisine without overdoing my sodium intake.

The good news is that research supports a reduction in appetite and preference for sodium as you get used to a lower sodium diet. Foods that you used to like might taste too salty after a month or two on a lower sodium diet. Now I don't really miss the sodium when I've substantially reduced salt as an ingredient. I do put the saltshaker on the table for my husband or guests and explain I am not in the least insulted to have them add salt to their food. Of course, since 90% of people eventually develop hypertension, it is not a bad thing to reduce the sodium intake of your friends and family!

There are foods I miss that just can't be made low sodium even by cooking them myself. I love feta cheese, black olives, pickles, and sauerkraut. I rarely use these items in cooking but if I do, I substantially reduce their amount in the recipe. I routinely either completely eliminate or drastically reduce the salt called for in recipes.

Note that there are some recipes that do not take well to drastic reduction of sodium. For example, yeast-risen breads rely on a specific amount of sodium to control the fermentation of the yeast. Too little sodium allows rapid fermentation and results in dough with poor texture. Be sure to use a recipe specially made for low sodium bread.

Many other recipes will turn out similarly if you drop or reduce salt as an ingredient. Table 23 shows how I modified the recipe for Chicken Tortilla Soup using lower sodium variations of ingredients. These easy changes dropped the sodium content over 80%. Remember, if you can't tolerate the degree of sodium reduction, you can always add a smidge of salt later.

However, there is no way to reduce the sodium content of a recipe you've already made.

Table 23. Example Modification of a Recipe—Chicken Tortilla Soup

Regular	Sodium (mg)	Lower Sodium Modifications	Sodium (mg)
2 T vegetable oil	0	Oil spray	0
1 32 oz. box Swanson chicken broth	2280	32 oz. of Swanson unsalted chicken stock	520
1 16 oz. can diced tomatoes	700	1 16 oz. can no salt added diced tomatoes	53
1 15 oz. can corn	630	2 cups frozen corn	16
12 oz. can Tyson chunk chicken	1500	2 cups chopped home-cooked chicken breast, low sodium brand	188
1 can Bush's black beans	1440	1 can Bush's lower sodium black beans	720
1 onion chopped	0	1 onion chopped	0
1 1.2 oz. package Ortega taco seasoning	2580	1 T cumin	0
		1 T chili powder	0
1 t salt	2000	1/8 t salt	250
½ cup fresh chopped cilantro	0	½ cup fresh chopped cilantro	0
4 oz. cheddar cheese shredded	704	2 oz. cheddar cheese, shredded	352
TOTAL sodium per recipe	**11,834**		2099
Sodium per 1 cup	**1183 mg**		**210 mg**

Directions: Sauté onion in pan for three minutes with oil spray. Add all other ingredients except cilantro and cheese in large pot on stove. Simmer for 30 minutes. Add cilantro and small amount of cheese on top before serving.

Eating a lower sodium diet does not need to be bland. Try spices or spice blends made without or low in sodium. You can buy these at the grocery store or make your own.

Shopping for Low Sodium Foods

One area of confusion is the belief that if you don't use the saltshaker at meals, you are eating a low sodium diet. In fact, only about 6-10% of sodium we eat is from salt added at the table. A similar amount is added in cooking. By far, the largest contributor to sodium intake in our diet, 75-80%, comes from restaurant and processed food.

The vast majority of the sodium we consume comes from foods that have already had substantial sodium added during processing or preparation. Historically, sodium was used for food preservation since salt inhibits bacterial growth. With refrigeration, this is less necessary. Contemporary reasons that manufacturers add sodium to foods include texture (*e.g.*, cheeses), a leavening agent (baking soda breads, cakes, cookies), fermentation (*e.g.*, sauerkraut or pickles), tenderness (meats and poultry), and taste. Salt is one of the least expensive taste enhancers, so it is used liberally in many foods. The amount of sodium added to meats or poultry can easily increase the sodium content six fold or more from the natural state. You can look at the label to see if sodium or brine has been used in processing of the meat or poultry.

There can be a wide variation in sodium content among brands of foods. Prepared salad dressings, for example, can vary from 50 to 500 mg per serving (see Table 24). You can see my recommended top limit, less than 120 mg, per serving in salad dressing in the bottom of the table. Get used to reading labels on foods at the grocery store. Labels are required to include sodium content in a serving. Make sure you notice what is called a serving as this may not be the amount you normally consume. In most supermarkets you can find lower sodium catsup, soy sauce, tomato sauces, and soups. My grocery store does not carry specialty items like low sodium pickles, microwave popcorn, or barbeque sauce, so I buy these on-line (e.g., http://healthyheartmarket.com/).

Cheeses range in sodium content by type with the highest usually in highly processed cheeses like American or those produced by brining like Feta (Table 25). Other high sodium cheeses include Blue, Romano, Roquefort, and Parmesan, while the lowest sodium cheeses tend to be Swiss, Gouda, Goat, Mozzarella, and cream cheese. Salt is used in the creation of cheese and as a preservative. Beware any cheese you see in a grocery store that does not need refrigeration as this likely means it contains a lot of salt!

Table 25 gives you a general idea of the sodium content of cheese, but this will vary by brand. A group of food scientists bought 650 Mozzarella cheese samples from grocery stores to analyze their sodium content. The samples ranged in actual sodium content from 129 to 250 mg per oz., an almost two fold difference [2]. Again, read the label to be sure what you are buying. My recommendation, as you shop, is to look for no more than 180 mg of sodium per 1 oz. serving for cheese.

Table 24. Example Sodium Content of Salad Dressings (2 T Serving)

Salad Dressing	Sodium (mg)
Lemon juice + oil (homemade)	0
Vino de Milo balsamic and olive dressing	55
Drew's roasted garlic and peppercorn	105
Marzetti strawberry chardonnay	140
Hidden Valley ranch	260
Newman's Own balsamic	290
Kraft thousand island	330
Wishbone Italian	340
Kraft roca blue cheese	380
Ken' Steakhouse Caesar	450
My recommended limit	**Less than 120 mg per 2 T**

Check the labels for brand-specific sodium content.

Table 25. Example Sodium Content of Cheese, 1 oz. serving

Cheese	Sodium (mg)
Swiss	54
Monterey jack	150
Ricotta (1/2 cup)	155
Cheddar	176
Mozzarella, part skim	175
Brie	178
Process American	263
Feta	316
Blue	395
Cottage cheese (1/2 cup)	400
Parmesan	454
My recommended limit	**Less than 180 mg per oz.**

*Data from National Dairy Council website

As we saw earlier, breads and cereals are the highest contributor to the sodium in the average American's diet. You can find lower sodium breads if you read the labels. Search for ones that contain less than 150 mg/slice. The lowest sodium choices for cereal are oatmeal that doesn't have added flavorings or shredded wheat brands (Table 26). Look for brands that have no more than 140 mg per oz. to keep your sodium intake low.

Table 26. Examples of the Sodium Content of Cereals (1 oz. Serving)

Cereal	Sodium (mg)
Quaker old fashioned or quick 1 minute oatmeal, ½ cup	0
Kellogg's Shredded Wheat, ¾ cup	0
Puffed Rice, 2 cups	2
Granola, no sodium added, ¼ cup	16
Kellogg's All Bran, ½ cup	75
Quaker organic maple and brown sugar, instant, 1 package	100
Quaker Life, ¾ cup	146
General Mills Cheerios, 1 cup	186
Quaker single-serve instant oatmeal	210
Corn Flakes, 1 cup	267
Post Grape Nuts, ½ cup	317
General Mills Wheat Chex, ¾ cup	395
My recommended limit	**Less than 140 mg/oz. (1 serving)**

The serving sizes vary in volume by type of cereal but are all equal to about 1 ounce.

Some companies produce low sodium versions of their products. For examples, see Table 27. As you can see, the regular product can contain up to 20 times more sodium as the lower sodium version. It can obviously make a big difference over the day if you use lower sodium versions of products.

Sodium content of prepared and frozen meals you pick up at the grocery store is likely very similar to that you find in a restaurant meal unless you find brands that purposely reduce the sodium levels. Table 28 lists some example single serving frozen entrées with their sodium content. You can see a wide variation between and within a brand. An exception is Healthy Choice brand, initiated in 1989 to provide consumers with frozen foods that fit into a healthy eating plan—it is lower in fat, calories, and sodium than comparable products. You can choose any Healthy Choice entrée and be sure that it is modest in sodium.

Traditional pasta sauces can be very high in sodium. However, there are many commercial versions that are reduced or low in sodium. Table 29 provides some examples. My recommendation is to look for pasta sauces that contain no more than 300 mg in a ½ cup serving. Of course, you could make much lower sodium pasta sauce yourself in a large batch and freeze it for later use. Use the no-sodium-added tomato products in the recipe.

Table 27. Sodium Content of Selected "Regular" and "Lower-Sodium" Versions of Food from Same Manufacturer

Product	Regular Version (mg)	Lower/No Salt-Added version (mg)
1 cup Swanson chicken stock	510	130
1 T Kikkoman soy sauce	920	575
1 T Heinz ketchup	160	25
2 slices Sara Lee honey ham	450	300
1 can Campbell's chicken with noodles soup	480	120
Nabisco Triscuit crackers, 28 g	160	50
Hunt's tomato sauce, ½ cup	820	40
Planter's mixed nuts, 28 g	95	50
Boar's Head roast beef, 2 oz.	230	40
Lucerne cottage cheese, ½ cup	440	45
Land-O-Lakes butter, 1 T	90	0

*From company websites

Table 28. Example Sodium Content of Boxed Frozen Meals

Item	Sodium per One Serving Entrée (mg)
Amy's Indian mattar paneer	780
Amy's light in sodium Indian mattar paneer	390
Amy's Thai stir fry	420
Banquet chicken pot pie	780
Banquet turkey and gravy	1070
Banquet Mexican style enchilada	1390
Healthy Choice grilled chicken marinara	550
Healthy Choice homestyle salisbury steak	543
Healthy Choice General Tso's spicy chicken	500
Kashi spicy bean enchiladas	600
Kashi pasta primavera	750
Kashi lemongrass coconut chicken	680

Kashi Mayan harvest bake	380
Stouffers Lean Cuisine five cheese rigatoni	650
Stouffers baked chicken breast for one	760
Stouffers beef stroganoff	990

Table 29. Examples of Sodium Content of Pasta Sauces (½ cup)

Item	Sodium (mg)
Enricos traditional pasta sauce, no salt added	35
White Oak Farm and Table tomato basil	200
Amy's light in sodium pasta sauce	290
Barillo marina, all natural	400
Prego Heart Smart traditional	430
Classico traditional sweet basil	470
Prego traditional	580
My recommended limit	**300 mg per ½ cup**

Determining Sodium Content from a Food Label

Sodium is one of only 12 nutrients that must be listed on a food label. The label provides the milligrams of sodium in one serving of the food. The size of one serving is defined at the top of the label (*e.g.*, ½ cup, 32 g) along with the number of servings in one package/container. Serving sizes may vary for foods within a category. For example, a serving size used on a label of Grape Nuts cereal is ½ cup, while a serving size of Corn Flakes is 1 cup. The serving size was designed to be the portion usually consumed, but you may normally eat more or less than this artificially defined serving size. The best way to determine this is by actually measuring the food after you have added it to your plate. Put the amount of cereal you usually eat into a bowl; pour this into a measuring cup. Once you have done this a few times, you will get a sense of your normal serving size.

In addition to milligrams of sodium per serving, the label will have the "% of DV". Labels use 2400 mg per day as the recommended daily value (DV). You can use this designation to find lower sodium foods. Look for foods that list 5%DV or less for sodium on the label; this represents 120 mg or less in a serving. On the other hand, avoid foods that provide 20%DV or more as this means it has at least 480 mg sodium in a serving. In addition to sodium, the label is required to list the grams of total fat, saturated and trans fat, carbohydrate and sugar, fiber, and protein. The milligrams of cholesterol as well as four micronutrients that are more often low in US diets (vitamin A, C, iron and calcium) are listed.

The FDA has proposed changes to the food label that are under review. This would be the first major revision to food labels since 1997. One change being considered is an update of the definition of a serving to be more similar to that which people really eat. The reality is that most people eat more than the currently listed serving size. The information about sodium is not expected to change in the new food label; both mg and %DV in a serving will be provided. Presently the potassium content of foods does not have to be listed. The FDA is considering adding this in the new food labels. This could be helpful for those with PA since low blood potassium is common.

Some foods have nutrition-related claims such as "low- fat" or "low-sodium." There are specific FDA definitions that must be met in order to use these claims. See Table 30 for definitions related to sodium claims.

Table 30. Interpreting Label Claims about Sodium

Sodium free	Less than 5 mg of sodium per serving
Very low sodium	35 mg of sodium per serving
Low sodium	140 mg of sodium or less per serving
Reduced or less sodium	At least 25% less per serving than regular
Light in sodium	50% less sodium than typical version

Although I would definitely choose a "reduced sodium" or "light in sodium" food over a similar one without this claim, beware that these foods could still have substantial sodium. I quickly picked up "reduced sodium" Dale's Steak Seasoning sauce at my grocery store but was shocked when I read the label at home showing it had 700 mg of sodium per tablespoon! Going on-line, I discovered the regular Dale's Steak Seasoning has 1220 mg sodium per tablespoon. So, although the label claim was accurate, this sauce provides more sodium than I want to consume. It is safest to consume "sodium free", "very low sodium" and "low sodium" foods.

Canned foods generally have sodium added during processing. Look for "no added sodium" or "low sodium" on the label or, better yet, use fresh food. For example, "no salt added" Hunt's canned tomato sauce has about 40 mg of sodium per cup compared to more than 800 mg in the same amount of "regular" tomato sauce. This could make a tremendous difference when used in a recipe.

Table 31 shows an example of the impact substituting lower sodium foods can have on your daily sodium intake. The lower sodium choices resulted in a sodium intake only one quarter as much as the reference day.

Table 31. Example of a One-day Diet with Substitutions to Reduce Sodium Intake

Rather than this	mg	Eat this	mg
Breakfast			
Oat ring cereal (1 cup)	284	Shredded wheat (1 cup)	0
Milk (1 cup)	127	Milk (1 cup)	127
English muffin (1)	293	Mixed grain bread, (1 slice)	140
Butter (2 t)	77	No-salt butter (2 t)	1
Lunch			
Bologna (2 slices)	578	Boar's Head low sodium roast beef (2 slices)	40
American cheese (1 oz.)	406	Swiss cheese (1 oz.)	74
Pumpernickel rye (2 slices)	364	Thin white bread (2 slices)	160
Horseradish, prepared (1 T)	198	Mayonnaise (1 T)	78
Snack			
Dry roasted peanuts (1/4 cup)	247	Unsalted peanuts (1/4 cup)	2
Dinner			
Commercial frozen lasagna (7.5 oz.)	671	Homemade lasagna made with lower sodium tomato sauce (7.5 oz.)	247
Carrots frozen in butter sauce (3.3 oz.)	350	Frozen, no sauce	43
Lettuce (1 cup)	0		0
French dressing (1 T.)	214	Vino de Milo balsamic and olive dressing (1 T)	28
Sandwich cookies (2)	96	Macaroons (2)	14
TOTAL	**3905 mg**		**954 mg**

USDA Home and Garden Bulletin 233

Pressure on Companies to Reduce Sodium Content in Prepared Foods

After reading this book, you might wonder why so much sodium is added to processed foods. The main reason manufacturers use so much salt is for taste, although sodium can also contribute to texture or improved preservation time of a food (salty ham or bacon can remain edible a long time). Salty is one of those inborn taste preferences that made sense when we lived in a world where sodium was scarce, but now it drives us to eat way too much when offered unlimited sources of sodium. You may worry that lower sodium consumption just won't be tolerable to you.

There is evidence that lower sodium products are acceptable to many consumers. One study comparing acceptability of foods that varied in sodium content concluded that a third or more reduction in sodium can be made without significantly affecting acceptance ratings [1]. So it may be easier than you think to reduce sodium intake.

Some companies have attempted to voluntarily reduce the sodium content of their products. For example, in the early 1980s companies like McDonald's, Quaker, and Campbell agreed to reduce sodium levels of their products. Modest changes were made in that the sodium content of representative products from McDonald's fell 9%, 23% for Quaker products, and 10% for Campbell's soups.

Unfortunately, most available evidence shows that little change has occurred in the sodium added to the majority of processed and restaurant foods. This is in spite of the fact that lower sodium foods are generally acceptable and that there is good evidence that this would be beneficial for public health. The Center for Science in the Public Interest began monitoring sodium content of 100 brand-name foods in 1983 and found the average sodium content decreased only 5% by 2004. Some individual foods even increased: for example, the sodium content of frozen dinners increased 82% over that period.

More recently, the New York City Health Department initiated the National Salt Reduction Initiative (NSRI) in 2008. At least 95 national, state and local health organizations joined this initiative to push a goal of reducing sodium content of restaurant and packaged food by 20% by 2014. The initiative worked with food industry representatives to set sodium targets for 62 packaged food and 25 restaurant food categories for 2012 and 2014. A set of about 27 restaurants, including Subway and Starbucks, as well as food manufacturers such as Kraft and Heinz, have currently committed to the initiative and have agreed to voluntarily reduce the sodium in their food products. Specifically, they agreed to reduce sodium levels of food categories in their line to NSRI targets. This means that some individual products the company sells could exceed the targets but others are lower so that the average sodium within the category reaches the goal.

The New York City Department of Health and Mental Hygiene developed (with funding from Centers for Disease Control and Prevention) an outstanding free database (see: www.MenuStat.org/) containing the nutritional content of foods served by 150 (as of the time of this writing) national restaurant chains. Although you could find all this information yourself from restaurants' websites, Menustat allows a one-stop-shop site where you can search by restaurant, by food type (*e.g.,* sandwiches), and nutrient. You can pull up similar foods in different restaurants to illustrate the differences in sodium content. The lists are updated each year to acknowledge the change in recipes used by the restaurants. This is an excellent free resource to locate lower sodium restaurant offerings at large chain restaurants.

The Center for Science in the Public Interest (CSPI) used the MenuStat database to assess whether restaurants have reduced sodium content of their offerings [14]. They compared seven food categories for 25 restaurant chains in 2012 to 2014. The results showed that there was no meaningful reduction in average sodium content across the food categories. The average sodium per food item in 2012 was 1266 mg; it was 1256 mg in 2014. The CSPI report compares the average sodium content across all items by restaurant. The restaurants with the highest average sodium were Applebee's, Chili's, IHOP, and Olive Garden where the average sodium per item was greater than 1500 mg, the recommended sodium intake for the entire day for those with hypertension. For comparison across restaurants, it is best to compare those of similar types. For example, compare Dunkin' Donuts with Starbucks or Burger King with Wendy's. The latter restaurant in both of those comparisons had lower average sodium in their offerings than the former. Of the restaurants monitored, Outback Steakhouse reduced sodium content the most, 9%, from 2012 to 2014.

Since changes in sodium are voluntary and there is no legislation about sodium content, it will be difficult to hold the companies to the NSRI agreement. The Institute of Medicine recommended in 2010 that policies mandating reductions in sodium in processed and restaurant foods be implemented, but this has not occurred.

Other countries have made bolder efforts to reduce population consumption of sodium. For example, in 2013, both Argentina and South Africa set mandatory sodium limits for categories of foods [13]. Although they are voluntary, the UK developed specific targets for 85 food categories in 2008. In addition, they implemented a traffic-light label system manufacturers are encouraged to use to indicate sodium content.

According to a survey of 1000 US adults done by the American Heart Association in 2013, 75% want less sodium in processed and restaurant foods, 58% have tried to reduce the amount of sodium in their diet, and 21% incorrectly believe there are already limits on how much sodium can be added to processed foods. However, until companies voluntarily reduce sodium content or we have regulations in the US that require change, you will need to be savvy on ways to select and prepare lower sodium foods.

Non-food sodium sources

Water contains some dissolved minerals, including sodium. Most public water or public health departments can provide you with the sodium content of your local municipal water—it is likely very modest. The US Environmental Protection Agency tested almost 1000 municipal water sources and found that 75% of them had less than 50 mg of sodium per liter (similar to a quart) of water. If you drank about eight glasses of water a day, this would translate to ingestion of less than 100 mg of sodium through drinking water. There are exceptions so check with your local public water department.

Those of us with well water must get it analyzed by a private company or local university extension office to know the quantity of minerals in our water. Note that well water may be "hard" in that it has a high proportion of minerals dissolved in it. This can leave scaling in pipes and plumbing fixtures as the minerals come out of solution. Hard water may also leave a residue on clothes after washing and make soap a less effective cleaner. You may be tempted to soften your water to fix this, but water softeners typically use salt so can dramatically increase the sodium in the water for drinking and cooking. The amount of sodium introduced to your water by a softening system depends on how hard your water was initially. The harder the water, the more sodium needs to be added to replace the dissolved minerals. The amount of sodium could be much more than that of untreated water. For example, one quart of softened water may have 200 mg of sodium, up to four times that of municipal water. There are water softeners that use potassium chloride instead of sodium chloride (salt), but it is much more expensive. My choice is to not use a water softener on our well water. You could also choose to soften your water to save your plumbing and clothes but bring home municipal or commercial water to drink.

Some medications, especially those used as antacids and laxatives, have enough added sodium that you could go over your goal. See Table 32 for sodium content of example nonprescription drugs.

Table 32. Sodium Content of Common Over-the-counter Drugs (one dose)

Drug	Sodium (mg)
Bromo-Seltzer	717
Alka-Seltzer	512
Rolaids	53
Metamucil Instant mix	250
Mylanta II	160

*from USDA Home and Garden Bulletin 233

Potassium

Potassium is a mineral required for life. It is crucial for heart and muscle contraction and plays an important role in blood pressure regulation. Population studies show that higher dietary potassium intake is generally associated with lower blood pressure. For example, a review that included 22 studies and almost 1900 people reported that increased potassium intake was associated with lower blood pressure in people with hypertension [6]. In fact, the highest potassium intake was associated with 24% lower risk of stroke. Many other studies support the fact that a higher potassium intake is cardiovascular protective.

The average potassium intake for adults in the US was 2640 mg per day in 2010, while the recommended intake is 4700 mg per day (Table 13). Less than 25% of men and 1% of women consumed this much potassium. Most men consume more potassium than women since men usually eat more food and calories. Many processed foods do not contain much potassium. Rich sources of potassium are fruits, vegetables, beans, dairy, coffee, fish, and unprocessed meat (Table 33). The average American gets about 20% of his/her potassium through fruits and vegetables, 11% from milk, 10% from meats and poultry, 10% from grain-based mixed dishes, and 7% from coffee and tea [37].

Remember that potassium content is currently not required to be on food labels. You can look up the potassium content of foods at websites like the SuperTracker program discussed earlier.

Table 33. Potassium Content of Example Potassium- Rich Foods

Food	Serving size	Potassium (mg)
V8 juice, low sodium	5.5 oz.	700
Potato, baked	1 medium	610
Yogurt	8 oz.	579
Banana	1	422
Tuna	3 oz.	484
Spinach	½ cup	419
Dried apricots	¼ cup	388
Non-fat milk	8 oz.	382
Tomato sauce	½ cup	380
Chicken	3 oz.	383
Beans	½ cup	355
Chicken	1 cup	343
Nuts (unsalted)	½ cup	300
Orange	1	237
Coffee	8 oz.	116
Tea	8 oz.	88

What role does potassium play in PA? As mentioned earlier in the diagnosis section, low blood potassium is a frequent consequence of PA because aldosterone increases excretion of this mineral. Low blood potassium causes some of the symptoms of PA, including muscle cramping. A low potassium intake could increase the likelihood of hypokalemia, so it makes sense to eat a diet rich in potassium. Although some PA patients might be prescribed potassium supplements to help boost blood potassium, I would not recommend potassium supplements unless they are prescribed and/or approved by your doctor.

A serious but rare potential side effect of spironolactone and eplerenone, key drugs already discussed for PA, is excessively high blood potassium. Since hyperkalemia can cause heart arrhythmia, taking a high dose potassium supplement in that situation could be deadly. Symptoms of hyperkalemia include stomach pain, weakness, and a feeling that the heart is beating irregularly. The amount of potassium in food is typically not enough to cause hyperkalemia, so stick to foods as sources of potassium unless your doctor recommends a supplement. Your medical team should regularly check your blood potassium, if a supplement is used, to insure that potassium does not get beyond the normal range.

Putting it together as DASH diet plan

US News and World Reports does annual ranking of the best colleges, doctors, and even diets. Its number one best overall diet for five years in a row through 2015 was the DASH diet. This diet was originally developed to reduce blood pressure; in fact, the acronym stands for "Dietary Approaches to Stop Hypertension," but it also has value for reducing blood lipids, losing weight, and reducing your risk of cancer. It is rich in vegetables, fruit, whole grains, nuts, beans, lean proteins, and low-fat dairy foods. This dietary pattern insures a high intake of vitamins that are sometimes low in the average American diet, like vitamin C and folate, as well as minerals potassium (K), magnesium (Mg), and calcium (Ca). The diet provides plenty of dietary fiber, known to improve intestinal regularity as well as aid in weight control. Fat is reduced to about 25% or less and saturated fat is kept to 7% of calories or lower while protein is slightly higher than average (approximately18%). A critical part of the plan is control of dietary sodium.

Carefully done studies using hypertensive patients or those with pre-hypertension (see Table 3) show a consistent and meaningful reduction in blood pressure in men and women of all races when they follow the DASH diet. The original research study published in 1997 using the DASH diet demonstrated a drop of 11.4 mm of systolic blood pressure of hypertensive individuals after eight weeks on the diet [5]. Older individuals, those with hypertension (especially resistant hypertension), and African American individuals were more responsive to the blood pressure lowering effect of the DASH diet than others [4]. The reductions observed are enough to cause a substantial reduction in risk for cardiovascular disease. For example, a statement from the American Heart Association indicates that a 3 mm drop in systolic blood pressure could lead to an 8% and 5% reduction in stroke and coronary heart disease mortality, respectively.

The original DASH diet contained about 3100 mg of sodium. The investigators were curious whether or not they would get an even greater benefit if sodium were reduced further. A second trial was initiated with three levels of dietary sodium: about 3300, 2500, or 1500 mg sodium per day. They determined that all reduced blood pressure but the best effect was using the lowest sodium DASH diet, 1500 mg [11].

The best resource for information and background of the DASH diet is at the National Heart, Lung, and Blood Institute (see: http://www.nhlbi.nih.gov/health/health-topics/topics/dash

Quick, think about how many servings of fruits and vegetables you ate yesterday. I am guessing that it doesn't hit the 8-10 goal as listed above for a 2000 calorie DASH diet (Table 34). In general, most people transitioning to the DASH diet will need to eat more fruits, vegetables, beans, and nuts than they usually do but less meat and sweets. Any rapid change in your normal diet is likely not sustainable and may cause digestive problems.

It is difficult to change your diet drastically and quickly. I recommend selecting 2-3 of the changes in Table 35 to try your first week. The next week, add a few more. Continue making changes until you reach the DASH goals. You are more likely to stick with the changes if you make them gradually. Remember to keep close track of your blood pressure and symptoms while you change your diet to note any connection.

Table 34 Number of Servings for Food Groups in the DASH Plan for a 1600 and 2000 Calories per Day Diet

Food Group	1600 Calories per Day	2000 Calories per Day	Definition of Serving
Grains	6	6-8	1 slice bread 1 oz. dry cereal ½ cup cooked rice, pasta, cereal
Lean meat, poultry, fish	3-4	5-7	1 oz. cooked 1 egg
Vegetables	3-4	4-5	1 cup leafy ½ cup cut up ½ cup juice
Fruit	4	4-5	1 whole ¼ cup dried ½ cup juice
Dairy, low fat or non-fat	2-3	2-3	1 cup milk or yogurt ½ cup cottage cheese 1.5 oz. cheese
Fats and oils	2	2-3	1 t. butter 1 t. oil 1 T. mayonnaise 2 T. salad dressing
Nuts, seeds, legumes	3-4/week	4-5/week	1/3 cup or 1.5 oz. nuts 2 T. peanut butter 2 T. or 1 oz. raw seeds ½ cup cooked legumes
Sweets and added sugars	3/week or less	5/week or less	

Table 35 Step-by-Step Strategies for the DASH Diet

Stop adding any salt at the table.
Add one more fruit and one more vegetable to lunch and dinner.
Use low sodium nuts as a snack in place of a sweet.
Increase the proportion of the "sodium-safer foods" listed in Table 16.
Buy whole grain breads and cereals.
Use dried fruit as a snack in place of a sweet.
Reduce the portion size of meat in your meal while expanding the whole grains (*e.g.*, brown rice).
Include a good protein source at each meal and snack, either a lean meat, fish, bean, poultry or low-fat dairy.
Substitute higher fat dairy foods with non-fat or low-fat.
Substitute whole grain pasta and rice for the white variety.
Drink water or flavored, no- calorie seltzer as beverage in place of soda.
Try some main dishes without meat but high in beans and whole grains.
Use fresh or frozen (no sauce) vegetables in place of canned.
Try lower sodium cheeses or butter.
Have DASH appropriate snacks ready for between meals (carrots, low sodium nuts, yogurt, dried fruits, low salt popcorn, low sodium rice cakes).

Select 2-3 strategies per week. Add more over time.

In addition to the above suggestions, all the earlier tips regarding selection of lower sodium foods apply to the DASH diet. That means not salting food at the table, altering recipes to include less salt, and buying foods at the grocery store to make low sodium eating and cooking easier. There are many good DASH recipe books and Internet sites available that will help you eat a lower sodium diet (Table 36). I use these resources for trying new recipes but more often simply modify the amount of salt or higher sodium ingredients and increase the fruits, vegetables, and grains in recipes my family and I already enjoyed.

Table 36. Example Internet Sources for Lower Sodium Recipes

Low Sodium
www.lowsodiumcooking.com
www.sodiumgirl.com
www.lowsodiumgourmet.com
http://www.heart.org/HEARTORG/GettingHealthy/NutritionCenter/Recipes/Heart-Healthy-Recipes-Responsive_UCM_465114_RecipeLanding.jsp
DASH Diet
https://healthyeating.nhlbi.nih.gov/default.aspx
http://dashdiet.org/dash_diet_recipes.asp
http://thedashdiet.net/
http://www.dashdietoregon.org/resources/recipes

You will likely get comfortable, over time, modifying the recipes. For example:

- Use only low sodium broths or soups, tomato sauce, vegetables, beans (all of these can be found in most major grocery stores).
- Use only lower sodium versions of sauces such as soy, teriyaki, catsup, BBQ sauce.
- Cut the salt amount in most recipes by 75-100%.
- Increase the use of spices.
- Buy no-salt seasoning blends or make your own.
- Increase the proportion of rice or whole grain pasta in a recipe.
- Use the lower sodium versions of products in a category for the recipe, e.g. pasta sauces, peanut butter, crackers, bread, cheese.
- Try some meat-free meals focused on beans as a protein source.

If you like to cook, you could prepare your own large quantities of lower sodium staples like pasta sauces, broths, and breads and freeze them in contains that are suitable for daily use. Or stock up on lower sodium products you purchase so you have them when you cook.

How can you check to see how close you are to the targets of the DASH diet? Using a table such as Table 37, you can list each food item you eat, check the definitions of the food groups for DASH (Table 34), and translate to the number of servings for each category in the row. At the end of the day, count up the servings for each column and determine how close you came to your goal. See an example of one-day diet with estimation of DASH food category servings in Table 38.

Table 37. Keeping Track of Compliance with DASH Diet

Item Example	Amount	Gr *	Veg	Fr	Milk	MPF	NSL	Fats	Sw
2 poached eggs						2			
1 slice toast		1							
1 t. butter								1	
8 oz. glass skim milk					1				

*Gr= grains, Veg = vegetables, Fr = fruits, MPF = meat, poultry, fish, NSL = nuts, seeds, legumes, Sw = sweets

Rather than going through more details of the DASH diet, I encourage you to download several free brochures describing use of the DASH diet as a way to reduce blood pressure at the National Heart Lung and Blood Institute   website (http://www.nhlbi.nih.gov/files/docs/public/heart/new_dash.pdf). Buy or borrow from the library some of the many good books already published with descriptions and recipes that fit a DASH diet approach. Food choices and recipes are modified to control the amount of sodium, fat, and sugar while liberally using fruits, whole grains, and vegetables.

Many PA patients are feeling better when following the DASH approach. You can find statements made by individuals who notice their symptoms (such as headache) coming back when they veer away from the DASH approach.

I do not consistently and perfectly following a DASH diet. Some days are closer to the DASH goals than others. Don't worry if you cannot achieve all of the dietary goals every day. Do the best you can with a special emphasis on reducing dietary sodium. You will likely feel better and have less risk of damage to your organs that comes from the combination of high blood aldosterone with sodium. Table 38 shows an example of a typical day's diet for me that roughly follows a DASH approach.

Table 38. A Typical Day Diet for Me Attempting a DASH Approach

Food	Sodium (mg)	Potassium (mg)	DASH Group
Breakfast			
16 oz. coffee	11	256	
½ cup oatmeal	0	140	1 Gr
1 cup skim milk	126	406	1 Milk
½ cup blueberries	4	65	1 Fr
½ cup homemade granola (no salt added)	1	206	1 Gr
Lunch			
2 cup fresh spinach	88	624	2 Veg
3.5 oz. chicken breast	63	167	3.5 MPF
1 piece bread	140	82	1 Gr
1 t no salt butter	0	0	1 Fat
¼ cup dried cranberries	0	70	1 Fr
1 apple	1	159	1 Fr
1 T dressing (lower sodium)	55	5	½ Fat
Snacks			
1/3 cup lightly salted roasted almonds	40	175	1 NSL
1 cup tea	5	66	
2 mini candy bars	85	85	1 Sw
Dinner			
1 cup homemade chili with beans and beef	250	625	2 MPF 1 NSL 2 Veg
1 piece bread	103	55	1 Gr
1 cup pineapple	1	175	2 Fr
1 cup frozen yogurt	116	257	1 Milk + 1 Sw
TOTAL	**1089 mg**	**3673 mg**	
DASH totals: 4 Gr, 2 Milk, 5 Fr, 4 Veg, 5.5 MPF, 2 NSL, 1.5 Fat, 2 Sw			

Gr= grains, Veg = vegetables, Fr = fruits, MPF = meat, poultry, fish, NSL = nuts, seeds, legumes, Sw = sweets

Caffeine, alcohol, supplements

Caffeine in doses of 200-300 mg can modestly, temporarily increase your blood pressure—usually 5-10 mm for an hour or so. However, most people adjust to daily caffeine so that their blood pressure changes less; they become accustomed to caffeine. You can test your own sensitivity by measuring your blood pressure (as described in earlier section) before and 30 minutes after ingesting caffeine. Coffee and some energy drinks contain high doses of caffeine, while tea and soft drinks are usually a more modest dose (Table 39). I have been a once-in-the-morning coffee drinker for many years. When I developed high blood pressure and did not know the cause, I began making and ordering cups with half decaffeinated and half regular coffee. I'm not sure that was necessary, but I am used to this now. I avoid energy drinks or medications with high caffeine.

Table 39. Caffeine Content of Common Foods and Beverages

Beverage	Caffeine (mg)
Starbucks tall coffee (12 oz.)	260
5-hour energy drink (1.9 oz.)	208
Monster energy drink (16 oz.)	160
McDonald's large coffee (16 oz.)	133
Red Bull (8.4 oz.)	80
Black tea (8 oz.)	30-80
Diet coke (12 oz.)	47
Starbucks decaffeinated coffee (16 oz.)	15-25
Herbal tea (8 oz.)	0
7 Up (12 oz.)	0

High alcohol consumption can increase high blood pressure but a modest intake of 1-2 drinks per day is not expected to influence blood pressure. Some medications should not be taken with alcohol, so read the patient information provided by the pharmacist on your prescriptions. For example, alcohol can reduce the effect of beta-adrenergic blockers, preventing the blood pressure reducing effect. On the other hand, alcohol can increase the effect of ACEi or diuretics to cause excessive drops in blood pressure with symptoms of dizziness or fainting.

Some dietary supplements are stimulants and therefore could increase your blood pressure. For example, bitter orange (citrus aurantium), ephedra (ma-huang), ginkgo (ginkgo biloboa), guarana (Paullinia cupana) are supplements that may increase your blood pressure. Other supplements could interact with your medications. It is important to tell your medical team what supplements you are taking. A brochure from the Agency for

Healthcare Research and Quality can be found for download on the Internet at: http://effectivehealthcare.ahrq.gov/ehc/products/223/1455/dietary-supplements-130509.pdf

Exercise

General physical activity for health

I am passionate about the importance of regular physical activity for health. As they say, if physical activity were a drug, everyone would want to take it. Increasing your fitness can reduce your risk of cardiovascular disease, diabetes, cognitive decline, osteoporosis (weak bones), stroke, and obesity. Plus, it just makes you feel good. Physical activity is an effective treatment for mild depression, and it is a stress reducer.

The national physical activity guidelines recommend that all adults get at least 150 minutes per week of moderate or 75 minutes of vigorous exercise per week. For example, this can translate to walking, swimming, or cycling at least 30 minutes, five days per week, or jogging for 25 minutes three times per week. This type of exercise, termed "aerobic," burns a good number of calories and contributes to a healthy heart.

In addition to aerobic exercise, muscle-strengthening exercise is recommended for all adults twice a week. This could include lifting weights in a gym, doing calisthenics, or taking an exercise class that involves weights. This type of exercise can help you avoid some of the drop in muscle mass that occurs due to aging and the reduction in bone mineral density that makes you vulnerable to osteoporosis.

Are there special considerations for physical activity for PA?

With all that said about the amazing benefits of being physically active, there is no evidence that physical activity will reduce your risk of PA or help you manage it better. The exception would be that your doctor may want you to limit vigorous physical activity if your blood pressure is very high or unstable or if you have diagnosed cardiovascular disease such as stroke, heart attack, pulmonary, or a metabolic disease like diabetes. In that case, you need to see your doctor before beginning any new exercise program.

Even if there is no evidence that regular exercise influences your PA, don't skip it (unless you have the limitations listed above). You want to get all those other benefits of physical activity for health and wellbeing. One safety tip, avoid breath holding during weight lifting, since this disproportionately increases blood pressure.

I have always been highly active and enjoy exercise. One of my favorite activities is road cycling. In fact, a few weeks before I had noted my first high blood pressure measurement, I had done my first 100-mile ride including over 5,000 feet of climbing. This was a struggle for me to complete, and in fact, both of my legs cramped at mile 100 such that I had to lie down until I recovered.

Did my developing PA have anything to do with the muscle cramps? There is no way to know but studies show that strenuous exercise increases the adrenal's secretion of aldosterone, especially if you are getting dehydrated. One effect of aldosterone is to increase loss of potassium. Was my blood potassium getting low, contributing to muscle cramps? I am curious but I will never know. Lots of people without PA get muscle cramps with vigorous exercise so it could be entirely unrelated for me.

I have been able to find very little information about exercise's influence on aldosterone (most I found were done in the 1980s), with nothing evaluating exercise in PA patients. Light exercise in neutral temperature environments did not increase aldosterone. However, strenuous exercise increased this hormone. For example, one of the few studies measuring the effect of exercise on aldosterone in "normal" people observed a 13-fold increase in aldosterone when subjects did strenuous exercise (80% of their maximum aerobic capacity) [53]. A rise in aldosterone in response to strenuous exercise makes sense since one of the adaptations to repeated sweat loss is to expand the blood volume to be better prepared for future exercise-induced dehydration. For this reason, exercising in a hot environment or when dehydrated increases aldosterone more than exercise in a cool environment. I do not know if aldosterone increases similarly in patients with PA when they exercise, but it makes sense that it would. Thus I now avoid highly strenuous activity that involves heavy sweating for a prolonged period. When I exercise, I am careful to drink fluids to avoid dehydration as this could further stimulate aldosterone (see Figure 3).

Drinking enough to prevent dehydration means that your body weight should not drop more than 1% over the exercise period. Any weight you lose during an exercise workout is due to water loss as you can't lose body fat that fast. For example, if you weigh 150 pounds, you should drink enough to avoid losing more than 1.5 pounds during exercise. You can check your weight shortly before and after the workout on a regular scale to get a sense of your dehydration.

The amount you need to drink during exercise will depend on many things, including how hard you are exercising, the temperature and humidity, your clothing, and how fit you are. As a ballpark plan, try to drink fluid regularly during the exercise workout—say every 15 minutes. If you are working out hard in a hot and humid environment, you might need to drink as much as 24 (3 cups) per hour. Most of us will need less than that to keep well hydrated since we are not likely working as hard as elite athletes. I shoot for drinking a whole 16 oz. bottle each hour when I am cycling.

Experiment by drinking what you think you need and then weighing yourself after the exercise to see how close your body weight is to the starting level. If you lost more than 1% of your original weight, try to drink more next time.

Note that it is also not good if you gain weight over an exercise workout. Excessive water retention during exercise can result in hyponatremia, a rare but possibly fatal condition when blood sodium drops too low. It occurs when someone is losing a lot of body sodium through sweat but replacing only water. This can dilute the blood sodium concentration to unusually low levels leading to serious symptoms. This condition occurs in a small percentage of marathon runners, for example. I only mention this rare condition in this book since I personally wonder whether treatment with eplerenone or spironolactone –drugs that reduce the retention of sodium-- combined with over-drinking water during exercise might increase the risk of hyponatremia. This is only speculation and I know of no case that has ever been reported. Symptoms of hyponatremia are dramatic and include dizziness, nausea, confusion, muscle cramps, and possible seizures. A sign that you may be losing too much sweat and drinking too much water would be a gain in body weight during exercise. My theoretical concern about this is another reason I, as a PA patient, will avoid extreme exercise where high sweat (and thus sodium) is lost. However, I will continue to exercise, in some way, almost every day.

Bottom line, I continue to exercise on a regular basis. It is good for my health, helps with weight control, and makes me feel better. However, my days of 100-mile bike rides are likely over. I usually do not exercise for longer than 1-2 hours, make sure I drink adequate water, and avoid exercising in the hot parts of the day.

Losing weight

It is difficult to change too many habits at once. So if weight loss makes sense for you, you might focus first on getting dietary sodium under control to improve your PA symptoms before you tackle any other dietary goals such as weight loss or blood lipid reduction. If you have multiple dietary issues to confront, it makes a lot of sense to involve a dietitian in your medical team. They can help you phase-in dietary changes over time.

There is no evidence, at this time, that body weight or amount of body fat is associated with risk of PA but it is associated with "essential" or "primary" hypertension. If you are overweight, losing weight will likely reduce your blood pressure if you have primary hypertension. In that condition, excess body fat increases inflammation and other factors that increase blood pressure.

Whole books are written on weight loss, and it is beyond the scope of this book to fully cover this topic. I have written a review posted in the references about dietary and exercise recommendations for body fat loss [64]. In fact, the DASH diet is fantastic for weight loss. The lower calories diet targets (1600 calories per day) listed in Table 34 would cause weight loss for most people. An appropriate goal is to reduce your calorie intake 300-500 calories per day while adding additional exercise.

If one of your goals is weight loss, I recommend that you include lean source of protein with each meal, including breakfast. This could be low or non-fat dairy like yogurt or milk, nuts, fish, poultry or lean beef. Consuming a rich protein source with each meal helps to increase your feeling of fullness. Research shows that people are better able to stick with a lower calorie diet when they eat protein throughout the day at modestly higher levels than is typical [64].

It also makes sense to reduce your intake of sugar and highly processed foods. These foods tend to make you want to eat more rather than satisfying you. They also contribute to an elevation in blood lipids, especially triglycerides. Insulin rises when you eat refined carbohydrates. Since insulin pushes potassium from the blood into cells, this could reduce the already low blood potassium lower in people with PA.

Exercise every day if you are trying to lose weight. It does not need to be strenuous, but the longer you do it, the better for calorie and fat burning. People who successfully lose weight and keep it off typically do up to an hour of exercise per day.

Chapter 9

CONTINUED LEARNING AND SHARING

There is new information being published every day about PA—causes, molecular mechanisms, treatment, and outcomes. So if you want to find out the latest information on this condition, you will need to continue to read beyond this book. This section provides some tips and some recommended resources for your continuing education.

Finding Information for the Public

There is much information available on the Internet, but it is not always easy to know which sites are trustworthy. Relying on US government websites is a good bet for finding quality information. The Office of Disease Prevention and Health Promotion coordinates the Healthfinder website (http://healthfinder.gov/). This website has information about everything from having a healthy pregnancy to parenting. You can find the latest health news that widely covers health topics. The "Health Conditions and Diseases" page provides tips and information for the top diseases in the US such as cancer, heart disease, and diabetes. This site can be useful if you would like additional information about common health conditions as well as some topics relevant to PA. For example, there is a link to quick tips on eating less sodium.

PA is not a topic covered within the Healthfinder portal but another government site, Medline Plus (http://www.nlm.nih.gov/medlineplus/) has relevant information. This site, described as "the National Institutes of Health's Web site for patients and their families and friends" is a portal produced and coordinated by the US National Library of Medicine. Reliable information on health and disease is presented in easy-to-read and understand manner. Provided website links have been evaluated for accuracy and reliability. The MedlinePlus articles are regularly updated with the last date up revision appearing on the bottom of the web page. To search for a topic, type key words into the search box or click on "health topics." You can also locate definitions of terms using the "medical dictionary" box on the home page or link to explore clinical trials on medical conditions.

Finding Research Articles

If you want to dig deeper than the information you can obtain in Medline or Healthfinder, you can also go to databases that focus on the original research papers from the medical literature such as PubMed (http://www.ncbi.nlm.nih.gov/pubmed/). This would be appropriate for individuals with good science backgrounds as some of the articles are written at a high scientific level. PubMed, a free search service managed by the US National Library of Medicine, has been in existence since 1996. It contains over 23 million references to biomedical and life science journal articles. You can search by topic or by author (see Table 40 for tips on searching) to find relevant articles.

Here are some steps and tips for searching with PubMed/Pub Med Central:

- Type a word or phrase into the search box.
- Use no punctuation.
- Make broader or more specific terms, as appropriate.
- Combine search terms with connector word: "AND", "OR", "NOT" (as upper case), as appropriate.
- Click on "search".
- Revise, as necessary.

Many of the listings will allow you to link to the website of the journal to view the full article but others will list only the reference (authors, journal title, date) with an abstract (summary) of the article. Some articles are protected by subscription and so are generally available at universities and large medical clinics but not to the general public. If you want to limit your search to only those articles that are available to you in full form for free, look to the left on the PubMed screen. Under "text availability" click on "full free text." By the way, don't even consider buying your own subscription. Most of these journals cost thousands of dollars per year for a subscription.

PubMed posts tutorials on searching their database including best ways to search for a specific topic. I recommend going to the "quick tour" videos on the PubMed page to get started.

You may be able to download the subscription-only articles through a local university or clinic electronic library. You might ask your doctor if he/she would find the article and share it with you. There is also a service through the National Library of Medicine called "Lonesome Doc" that will connect you to a library that has full access to the article. Use of Lonesome Doc is free, but you may have to pay the connecting library for the article. Finally, most scientific papers provide the email address of the first author. You can try emailing the author to ask for a copy of the paper.

PubMed Central was developed by the National Library of Medicine in 2000 as a free archive of biomedical and life science publications. Thus free access to the over three million journal articles in PubMed Central is available to everyone. You can get to PubMed Central by going to PubMed and selecting "PMC" from the drop down menu on the left of the search box. You may be surprised to see all the articles available to you.

Once you get a list of references (provided as 20 per page with most recently published first) that fit your search, click on any one of them to get to read the full article. To save a copy, click on "PDF" (you must have downloaded the free Adobe Reader software from Adobe in order to do this step). You will notice that a short list of "related citations" will appear next to the article. This is another way to locate additional similar research publications.

You can sign up for notification of newly published articles by registering (for free) for "My NCBI" (National Center for Biotechnology Information) at the top right of the PubMed webpage. After you create a user ID and password, you can create various searches (*e.g.*, "primary aldosteronism" or "resistant hypertension AND sodium"). These "email alerts" sent to your email either daily, weekly, or monthly, depending on how you set it up, will contain a list of new articles related to your search term(s).

Of course, these articles will be written at a high level and may be difficult to understand. You might ask someone with a bio-science or medical background to help you interpret them.

Although I do not use it often, you can also search Google Scholar (https://scholar.google.com/) to find resources on any topic. In addition to containing links to published research articles, Google Scholar may list theses/dissertations and technical reports on various topics. A green triangle indicates that you can find the resource for free.

Once you have investigated research related to PA, you will find there is a subset of authors that come up again and again. You can search for publications by any particular author using the search databases described above. For example, find out the most recent published articles by John W.

Funder by typing in "funder jw", last name followed by initials without punctuation. Be as specific as possible with the author name, using middle initials if you know them. This is effective if the name is uncommon but you will get a lot of articles to look through if you search for "wang l," for example.

There are some clinics or research groups that focus on PA. They continue to collect data on patients and experiment with new treatments. For example, the German Conn's Registry (http://www.conn-register.de/) was established in 2006 in Munich. This center collects data from multiple German clinics about PA patients. Their goal is to improve diagnosis, treatment, and care of PA patients and to develop standards for use by other clinics. Many publications have come out of this registry. Tip: access this site using Google Chrome web browser since it will offer you a choice to "translate" the page from German to English.

Websites Related to PA

An interesting blog from JaneRay1940, an individual who went through adrenalectomy can be found at https://waywardbus.wordpress.com/. The author provides various useful links to resources for PA patients as well as detailed descriptions of her personal journey with PA.

Another website was created by Carole A. Langrall, who was diagnosed with PA in 2008 (http://hyperaldosteronism.blogspot.com/). She describes going through diagnostic testing and treatment as adrenalectomy. The writer has very useful practical tips about living with PA, working with doctors, and preparing for procedures.

The National Adrenal Diseases Foundation (NADF) website (http://www.nadf.us/) has a downloadable fact sheet on PA as well as some patient questions with responses from the NADF medical director.

I developed a website to highlight recent developments on primary aldosteronism. I intend to use this site to post summaries of some of the new research publications I read related to this condition (https://primaryaldosteronism.wordpress.com/).

Connecting with Other PA Patients

A highly useful website is the Yahoo group on primary aldosteronism (https://groups.yahoo.com/neo/groups/hyperaldosteronism/info). This site has over 1,000 registered members (although most do not appear to be regularly active). People post questions or comments on this site that is open only to those approved by the moderator. However, this is easily done once you have set up a Yahoo account with username and password. You will be required to send an inquiry to the "hyperaldosteronism group" moderator explaining why you would like to join. Following approval, you can post your own "story," read the stories of others, read the articles that have been posted in the group page, and read or post emails to the group.

There are fascinating questions and responses from people with PA, some who have apparently been involved in this site for a long time. The best part about the group is that a semi-retired physician, Dr. Clarence Grim, is the moderator and daily provides answers and feedback to the queries posted. Dr. Grim worked with Dr. Conn who, as you remember, discovered and provided a name for this condition. Dr. Grim has worked for over 50 years in endocrinology with special emphasis on PA. He provides useful, short responses to most questions, every day, and participates in the discussions on the Yahoo group site. I believe this is an incredible public service. If you desire more individual attention, Dr. Grim will agree to consult individually with you and your medical team for a fee. Dr. Grim has also set up some surveys to collect information from members to look for commonalities and issues experienced by members. It is not a formal research "registry" that is carefully collected and managed but it is a free, highly accessible resource to understand what other PA patients have experienced.

See this quote from someone who hired Dr. Grim as a consultant to help her medical team:

> *I absolutely credit him with saving my life. I could not have been very far away from a major stroke until he entered the picture. Even after getting the CT scan, to confirm my diagnosis, none of my doctors knew what to do with the information except prescribe spiro[nolactone]. The absolute importance of a low sodium diet was never stressed, except by Dr. Grim, and the low sodium diet is what makes all the difference. He guided my doctors through the process of getting rid of most of my BP meds, which they would have been far too cautious to do on their own. (Dianne)*

I found the organization of the Yahoo group documents awkward; you will have to do significant searching for specific topics. However, I have learned an incredible amount by reading and posting on this group site. It is, to me, a wonderful use of the Internet to share knowledge and experiences. Some of the patients who post are highly knowledgeable about PA. Realize that nothing that is posted is verified for accuracy, but usually other members will clarify something that does not appear correct.

Another patient portal that includes patients with PA is "Inspire" (www.inspire.com). This portal is a place for patients with a wide variety of conditions to share and communicate with one another. The platform used for interaction on this site is much superior, in my opinion, to the Yahoo site. You will need to set up an account and indicate which conditions you are interested in. You can either go to the site to see what has been posted or ask to be sent a weekly digest that summarizes active and new postings under the condition of interest. I found some very interesting but a modest number of posts related to PA. I believe that most PA patients find their way to the Yahoo group site since there is more activity and more members.

I also came across another website forum for PA patients at www.mdjunction.com. You can search for questions posted about PA or post your own questions to the "Conn's Syndrome Discussions." The site appears to have much less traffic than the Yahoo site but has a very nice interface with strong possibilities. Check it out.

Family and Friends

Friends and family can provide powerful support for you in managing PA. I was very appreciative of my husband's help when I was scared during my erratic very high blood pressure bouts and that he was willing to listen as I sought to understand what was happening to me. It can be very frustrating and alarming to have unusual symptoms without diagnosis. Talking to someone close may help.

Your partner or spouse can provide important information about signs of your disease. In other words, do you look pale, snore or stop breathing at night, appear short of breath with modest activity? Since they see you regularly, spouses and partners may notice important signs that should be shared with your medical team.

On the other hand, irritation or impatience from partners or spouses may occur. For example, you might repeatedly wake them at night when you get up multiple times to empty your bladder. Your fatigue could keep you from doing activities together; medications can influence your libido. The new expense of medical tests, medications, unique foods can add to family stress. The new stress of a disease can bring partners closer or break them apart, depending on how they handle it.

Although I don't know of any local PA support groups, it is possible they exist through your medical clinic. Ask your doctor. As mentioned in the last section, there are on-line support groups (*e.g.*, Yahoo, Inspire) that can provide ideas for coping with unsupportive friends or family.

It could be that your spouse or partner does most of the food shopping and/or cooking in your household. If so, it is critical that you involve them in learning more about the disease and the importance of dietary changes.

As the primary food shopper and cook in my own home, it is easier to ensure that meals fit my PA management program. However, the fact that my husband is agreeable to new recipes with less salt and more vegetables helps me stick with my plan. It would be much more difficult if I had to constantly watch him eating things that I could not.

Although I can understand some people remaining private, I share with friends that I have PA. I believe it is valuable for them to understand why I may avoid certain restaurants or not eat something they might serve for dinner.

Some friends may not want to know the details of your condition. Have a short explanation that will provide just the basics. For example, "I have a hormonal condition that requires daily medication and a low salt diet" or "I have high blood pressure caused by a hormonal imbalance that is controlled through diet and medication" may be all they need.

Chapter 10

FINAL WORDS

My goal with this book is to provide information that will be useful to those who have been diagnosed with or suspected to have PA. Although the title of the book makes it sound like a promise that you will be "cured," the reality is that only those who have an adrenalectomy may truly move forward without the disease. If you have adrenal hyperplasia in both adrenals or do not want to undergo surgery even though eligible, your disease can likely be well managed or dramatically improved with appropriate medications and diet. This has been my experience.

Many scientists and clinicians write that PA is "the most curable type of hypertension." Unfortunately, it is also one of the least correctly diagnosed. My intention is that this book push society in the direction of more awareness and appropriate treatment of this condition resulting in a longer and better quality life. My hope is that this book has helped most readers in some way and expands the recognition of PA as a serious but treatable condition.

CHECK LIST FOR PRIMARY ALDOSTERONISM

Do you have <u>several</u> of these symptoms?

- Fatigue
- Headache
- Muscle weakness or cramps
- Numbness
- Polyuria (excessive urination), especially at night
- Polydipsia (excessive thirst)

AND <u>one</u> of these applies to you:

- Blood pressure verified as greater than 160/100 mm
- You are on at least three medications without achieving blood pressure target
- Hypokalemia (low blood potassium, usually considered less than 3.5 mmol/L)
- Hypertension with adrenal mass (e.g. discovered via CT or other imaging)
- Hypertension with family history of early onset hypertension or stroke less than 40 years of age
- Patients with a first-degree relative (e.g. father/mother, sibling, offspring) with PA

Then, ask your doctor about primary aldosteronism.

GLOSSARY

For terms not found, go to the Medline medical dictionary:
http://www.nlm.nih.gov/medlineplus/mplusdictionary.html

Adenoma- benign (not cancerous) tumor in a gland

ACE- Angiotensin Converting Enzyme, converts angiotensin I to angiotensin II

ACEi- angiotensin converting enzyme inhibitor drug

ACTH- adrenocorticotropic hormone, produced by the pituitary gland, stimulates the adrenal gland

Adrenal gland- glands above kidney that secrete a variety of hormones including mineralocorticoids (e.g. aldosterone), glucocorticoids (e.g. cortisol), and catecholamines (e.g. epinephrine)

Adrenalectomy- surgical removal of the adrenal gland

Aldosterone- a corticosteroid hormone produced by the adrenal gland, increases kidney reabsorption of water and sodium, elevated secretion in aldosteronism

Angiogram- radiographic view of an artery or arteries after injecting a substance viewable by the radiograph

Angioplasty- use of catheter balloon or surgery to open a narrowed artery

Angiotensin- protein that, when activated to angiotensin II, stimulates the secretion of aldosterone in adrenal gland

Angiotensinogen- precursor for angiotensin, forms angiotensin I when acted on by ACE

APA- aldosterone-producing adenoma, most common form of primary aldosteronism, adenoma on one or both adrenal glands

ARB- angiotensin receptor blocker drug

ARR- aldosterone renin ratio, used as part of diagnosis of primary aldosteronism

Arrhythmia- abnormal electrical conduction and contraction of the heart

Atherosclerosis- artery walls thicken as a result of infiltration of immune cells and lipids; blood vessel diameter is reduced allowing less blood flow

Atrial fibrillation- the most common arrhythmia in primary aldosteronism, rapid and uncoordinated contraction of the upper chambers of the heart

Beta-blocker- drugs that block the beta receptors for catecholamines in the blood vessels, heart and brain; cause slower heart rate and vasodilation

BUN- blood urea nitrogen, urea is produced in the liver and excreted by the kidney

Calcium channel blocker- drugs that bind to calcium channels in the heart and muscle cells; cause vasodilation and slower heart rate

Captopril challenge- test used to diagnose PA; involves ingestion of captopril and measurement of aldosterone response

Conn's syndrome-another term used to refer to primary aldosteronism, particularly aldosterone-producing adenoma

CT scan- imaging technique used to look at cross sectional pictures of the body; abdominal CT scan used to look for adrenal tumors

Cushings syndrome- a disease defined by over-release of ACTH from the pituitary gland that stimulates high secretion of cortisol from the adrenal gland

DASH- dietary approach to stop hypertension; diet recommending high fruit, vegetable, legume, dairy, lean protein food sources that results in low sodium and high potassium intake

Diastolic blood pressure- the second and lower number when blood pressure measured; the pressure against the vessel walls during the period when no blood is being ejected from the heart into the circulatory system

Diuretic-drugs that increase water and sodium loss from body by increasing urine production; some also increase loss of body potassium

Echocardiogram- ultrasound test that uses sound waves to produce images of the heart as it contracts

Endocrinologist- doctors who specialize in diseases related to the glands and hormones

Eplerenone- a mineralocorticoid receptor antagonist medication used to treat primary aldosteronism

Fibrosis- organ tissue becomes thick and often less functional

Genetic mutation- a change in a gene that can result in expression of abnormal proteins; changes can be passed to offspring

Glomerular filtration rate- test to check how well the kidneys are functioning; specifically estimates the amount of blood that goes through the kidney glomeruli per minute; low rates can be associated with kidney disease

GRA- glucocorticoid- remediable aldosteronism; a form of genetic PA

Gynecomastia- growth of breasts in men

Half- life- amount of time for half of a drug to be broken down

Hirsuitism- excessive hair growth on a woman's body or face

Hyperkalemia- excessively high blood potassium, often defined as > 6.0 mmol/L but may vary by laboratory

Hypertension- high blood pressure; typically considered when blood pressure great than 140/90 mm Hg if less than 60 years, diabetic or with kidney disease; greater than 150/90 if older than 60 years

Hypertrophy- increase in volume of an organ or tissue; e.g. left ventricular hypertrophy

Hypokalemia- low blood potassium, typically defined as < 3.5 mmol/L but may vary by laboratory

Hyponatremia- low blood sodium

IHA- idiopathic hyperaldosteronism, hyperplasia of adrenal cells that secrete excess aldosterone

Inflammation- immune system response to injury or various infectious agents or chemicals; acute (short-term) inflammation causes swelling, pain and loss of function with the attempt to resolve the injury or pathogen; chronic inflammation (long-term) can affect destruction or healing of tissue

Insulin sensitivity- degree that body cells respond normally to insulin; in insulin insensitive conditions insulin is present but less effective than normal

JNC8- 8th Joint National Committee; developed latest hypertension guidelines for medial professionals

Laparoscopic surgery- surgery performed via insertion of a tube with blade into small incisions; typically is less invasive and involves smaller incision than traditional "open" surgery

Left ventricular hypertrophy (LVH)- enlargement of the muscle tissue of the lower chamber of the left side of the heart

Lipids- fats, typically referring to blood fats such as triglyceride and cholesterol

Metabolites-chemical produced during metabolism, in drug metabolism refers to the breakdown products when the drug is broken down in the body

Mineralocorticoid- steroid structure hormones that influence salt and water balances; aldosterone is an example secreted by the adrenal cortex

Glossary

Mineralocorticoid receptor- receptor for mineralocorticoid (such as aldosterone) attachment on cell; stimulates signals that act on the cell

MRI- magnetic resonance imaging; uses magnetic field with radio frequency pulses to provide images of organs

Myocardial infarction- heart attack, typically due to inadequate blood flow and oxygen delivery in the heart arteries; causes death of some of the heart cells

Naturesis- excretion of sodium in the urine

Nephrons- filtering units of the kidney

Nephrologist- doctor who specializes in diseases of the kidney

NSAID- nonsteroidal anti-inflammatory drug, used for reduction of pain or fever (examples include Naproxen, Ibuprofen)

Obstructive sleep apnea- interruption of breathing during sleep that can reduce blood oxygen and arousal

Osteopenia- moderate reduction in bone volume and strength

Osteoporosis- substantial reduction in bone volume and mineral density resulting in increased risk of fracture

PAC- plasma aldosterone concentration

Parathyroid hormone (PTH)-hormone secreted by the parathyroid gland; involved in the metabolism of calcium and phosphorous in the body

Pericardial effusion- build- up of fluid outside the heart

Pheochromocytoma- rare tumor in the adrenal gland that results in excessive secretion of epinephrine (adrenaline) and norepinephrine; one cause of secondary hypertension

Pituitary gland- endocrine gland at the base of the brain that secretes a variety of hormones including those that regulate growth, blood pressure, metabolism, temperature regulation, and menstrual cycle/pregnancy (e.g. growth hormone, thyroid- stimulating hormone, ACTH, prolactin, luteinizing hormone, anti-diuretic hormone)

Polydipsia- excessive thirst

Polyuria- excessive urination; especially common at night for PA patients

Potassium- mineral that is required in the diet; has important roles in muscle and heart function as well as body water balance

PRA- plasma renin activity

Prehypertension- blood pressure that is higher than normal but not to the hypertensive level; American Heart Association defines this as 120-139 mm systolic or 80-89 mm diastolic blood pressure

Primary aldosteronism- disease characterized by excessive production and secretion of aldosterone from the adrenal gland; results in excess sodium and water retention; most common cause of secondary hypertension

Primary hypertension (also called "essential hypertension")- high blood pressure due to no clear-cut cause but typically associated with obesity, poor diet, sedentary lifestyle, or genetics

Prolactin- hormone produced by the pituitary gland; stimulates breast development and milk production

PubMed- Internet search engine for articles in the biomedical literature

RAAS- Renin, angiotensin, aldosterone system

Renal artery stenosis- narrowing of the arteries leading to the kidney; a cause of secondary hypertension

Renin-enzyme secreted by the kidney when low blood volume or low blood sodium is sensed; breaks down angiotensinogen to angiotensin I in the bloodstream

Glossary

Resistant hypertension- blood pressure that does not achieve target in spite of three or more medications

Secondary hypertension- high blood pressure caused by another medical condition

Signs- evidence of medical issue or disease that is seen by an observer (e.g. pale face, excessive sweating)

Sodium- mineral required in the diet; sodium has important roles in nerve and muscle function as well as body water balance

Somatic mutation- change in the DNA of a cell after birth; often caused by environmental stresses such as radiation or chemicals; genetic change not passed onto off-spring

Spironolactone- a mineralocorticoid receptor antagonist medication used to treat primary aldosteronism

Stroke- rupture or obstruction of the arteries to the brain resulting in death of some brain cells from low blood oxygen

Sympathetic drive- magnitude of activation of the sympathetic nervous system; involved with preparing the body to react to stress or emergency; increases heart rate and blood pressure as well as other physiological changes

Symptoms- subjective evidence of medical issue or disease experienced by the individual (e.g. dizzy)

Systolic blood pressure- blood pressure during period that the ventricles, lower chambers of the heart, are contracting and ejecting blood into the circulation; the first and higher of the two numbers that are typically given for blood pressure

Thrombosis- blood clot

Ultrasound- Imaging technique that involves use of sound waves; renal artery duplex is an example medical test that utilizes ultrasound

Vasoconstriction- narrowing of the diameter of the blood arteries and arterioles

REFERENCES

1. Adams SO, O Maller, AV Cardello. 1995 Consumer acceptance of foods lower in sodium. Journal of the American Dietetic Association. 95:447-453.

2. Agarwal S, D McCoy, W Graves, PD Gerard, S Clark. 2011 Sodium content in retail Cheddar, Mozzarella, and process cheeses varies considerably in the United States. Journal of Dairy Science. 94:1605-1615.

3. Amar L, M Azizi, J Menard, S Peyrard, PF Plouin. 2013 Sequential comparison of aldosterone synthase inhibition and mineralocorticoid blockade in patients with primary aldosteronism. Journal of Hypertension. 31:624-629.

4. Appel LJ. 2014 Reducing sodium intake to prevent stroke: time for action, not hesitation. Stroke. 45:909-911.

5. Appel LJ, MW Brands, SR Daniels, N Karanja, PJ Elmer, FM Sacks. 2006 Dietary approaches to prevent and treat hypertension. Hypertension. 47:296-308.

6. Arburto NJ, S Hanson, H Gutierrez, L Hooper, P Elliott, FP Cappuccio. 2013 Effect of increased potassium intake on cardiovascular risk factors and disease: systematic review and meta-analysis. British Medical Journal. Apr 3.

7. Bender SB, AP McGraw, IZ Jaffe, JR Sowers. 2013 Mineralocorticoid receptor-mediated vascular insulin resistance. Diabetes. 63:313-319.

8. Catena C, G Colussi, E Nadalini et al. 2008 Cardiovascular outcomes in patients with primary aldosteronism after treatment. Archives of Internal Medicine. 168:80-85.

9. Catena C, G Colussi, L Sechi. 2013 Aldosterone, organ damage and dietary salt. Clinical and Experimental Pharmacology and Physiology. 40:922-928.

10. Catena C G Colussi, F Nait, F Martinis, F Pezzutto, LA Sechi 2014 Aldosterone and the heart: still an unresolved issue? Frontiers in Endocrinology 5, article 168.

11. Champagne CM 2006 Dietary interventions on blood pressure: the

Dietary Approaches to Stop Hypertension (DASH) Trials. Nutrition Reviews. 64:S53-S56.

12. Champagne CM, GA Bray, AA Kurtz, JB Monteiro, E Tucker, J Volaufova et al. 2002 Energy intake and energy expenditure: a controlled study comparing dietitians and non-dietitians. Journal of American Dietetic Association. 102:1428-1432.

13. Center for Disease Control and Prevention. 2012 Vital signs: food categories contributing the most to sodium consumption—United States, 2007-2008, MMWR. 61:92-98.

14. Center for Science in the Public Interest. 2014 Restaurants can't shake the salt. http://cspinet.org/images/salt-report-draft.pdf.

15. Colussi G, C Catena, LA Sechi. 2013 Spironolactone, eplerenone and the new aldosterone blockers in endocrine and primary hypertension. Journal of Hypertension. 31:3-15.

16. Cook NR, JA Cutler, E Obarzanek, JE Buring, KM Rexrode, SK Kumanyika et al. 2007 Long term effects of dietary sodium reduction on cardiovascular disease outcomes: observational follow-up of the trials of hypertension prevention (TOHP) British Medical Journal. April 28:885-888.

17. Cupp M. 2013 The "triple whammy" Pharmacist's Letter/Prescriber's Letter. April 2013.

18. Dhanjai TS, DG Beevers. 2008 Delay in the diagnosis of Conn's Syndrome: a single-center experience over 30 years. Hypertension. 52:e22.

19. Du Cailar G, P Fesler, J Ribstein, A Mimran. 2010 Dietary sodium, aldosterone and left ventricular mass changes during long-term inhibition of the renin-angiotensin system. Hypertension. 56:865-870.

20. Eckel RH, JM Jakicic, JD Ard, VS Hubbard, JM de Jesus, IM Lee et al. 2013 AHA/ACC Guideline on lifestyle management to reduce cardiovascular risk. Circulation. 129:S1-S45.

21. Fischer E, F Beuschlein, M Bidlingmaier, M Reinchke. 2011 Commentary on the Endocrine Society practice guidelines: consequences of adjustment of antihypertensive medication in

screening of primary aldosteronism. Reviews in Endocrinology and Metabolic Disorders. 12 43-48.

22. Fischer E, F Beuschlein, C Degenhart, P Jung, M Bidlingmaier, M Reincke. 2012 Spontaneous remission of idiopathic aldosteronism after long-term treatment with spironolactone: results from the German Conn's registry. Clinical Endocrinology. 76:473-477.

23. Fox CS, MG Larson, SJ Swang, EP Leip, N Rifai, D Levy et al. 2006 Cross-sectional relations of serum aldosterone and urine sodium excretion to urinary albumin excretion in a community-based sample. Kidney International. 69:2064-2069.

24. Francis J, RM Weiss, SG Wei, AK Johnson, TG Beltz, K Zimmerman. 2001 Central mineralocorticoid receptor blockade improves volume regulation and reduces sympathetic drive in heart failure. American Journal Physiology: Heart Circulation 281:H2241-H2251.

25. Francesconi RP, MN Sawka, KB Pandolf. 1983 Hypohydration and heat acclimation: plasma renin and aldosterone during exercise. Journal of Applied Physiology Respiratory Environmental and Exercise Physiology. 55:1790-1794.

26. Funder JW. 2012 Primary aldosteronism: clinical lateralization and costs. Journal of Clinical Endocrinology and Metabolism. 97:3450-3452.

27. Funder JW. 2014 Primary aldosteronism and salt. Pfugers Archives European Journal of Physiology. 467:587-594.

28. Funder JW, RM Carey, C Fardella et al. 2008 Case detection, diagnosis, and treatment of patients with primary aldosteronism: an Endocrine Society clinical practice guideline. Journal of Clinical Endocrinology and Metabolism. 93:3266-3281.

29. Gaddam K, E Pimenta, SJ Thomas, SS Cofield, S Oparil, SM Harding et al. 2010 Spironolactone reduces severity of obstructive sleep apnea in patients with resistant hypertension: a preliminary report. Journal of Human Hypertension. 24:532-537.

30. Gallay BJ, S Ahmad, L Xu, B Toivola, R Davidson. 2001 Screening for primary aldosteronism without discontinuing hypertensive medications: plasma aldosterone-renin ratio. American Journal of Kidney Diseases. 37:699-705.

31. Gonzaga CC, KK Gaddam, MI Ahmed, E Pimenta, SJ Thomas, SM Harding et al. 2010 Severity of obstructive sleep apnea is related to aldosterone status in subjects with resistant hypertension. Journal of Clinical Sleep Medicine. 6:363-368.

32. Gravez B, A Targus, F Jaisser. 2013 Mineralocorticoid receptor and cardiac arrhythmia. Clinical and Experimental Pharmacology and Physiology. 40:910-915.

33. Grim CE. 2004 Evolution of diagnostic criteria for primary aldosteronism: why is it more common in "drug-resistant" hypertension today? Current Hypertension Reports. 6:485-492.

34. Hanusch FM, E Fischer, K Lang, S Diederich, S Endres, B Allolio et al. 2014 Sleep quality in patients with primary aldosteronism. Hormones. 13:57-64.

35. He FJ, GA MacGregor. 2002 Effect of modest salt reduction on blood pressure: a meta-analysis of randomized trials. Implications for public health. Journal of Human Hypertension. 16:761-770.

36. Hlavacova N, J Bakos, D Jezova. 2010 Eplerenone, a selective mineralocorticoid receptor blocker, exerts anxiolytic effects accompanied by changes in stress hormone release. Journal of Psychopharmacology. 24:779-786.

37. Hoy MK, JD Goldman. 2012 Potassium intake of the U.S. Population, NHANES 2009-2010. Food Surveys Research Group Dietary Data Brief #10, USDA.

38. Hutchins R, AJ Vier, SL Sheridan, MP Pignone. 2015 Quantifying the utility of taking pills for cardiovascular prevention. Circulation Cardiovascular Quality Outcomes. 8(2):155-163.

39. Indra T, R Holaj, B Strauch, et al. 2014 Long-term effects of adrenalectomy or spironolactone on blood pressure control and regression of left ventricle hypertrophy in patients with primary aldosteronism. Journal of the Renin-Angiotensin- Aldosterone System. Epub ahead of print.

40. Institute of Medicine. 2013 Sodium Intake in Populations: Assessment of Evidence. Washington DC: National Academies Press.

References

41. Intersalt Cooperative Research Group. 1988 INTERSALT: an international study of electrolyte excretion and blood pressure: results for 24 h urinary sodium and potassium excretion. British Medical Journal 197: 319-328.

42. James, PA, Oparil S, BL Carter et al. 2014. 2014 evidence-based guideline for the management of high blood pressure in adults: report form the panel members appointed to the eighth joint national committee (JNC8) JAMA. 311:507-520.

43. Jin J. 2014 Patient page: New guidelines for treatment of high blood pressure in adults. JAMA. 311:538.

44. Jin Y, T Kuznetsova, M Maillard, T Richart, L Thijs, M Bochud, et al. 2009 Independent relations of left ventricular structure with the 24-hour urinary excretion of sodium and aldosterone Hypertension. 54:489-495.

45. Karagiannis A, K Tziomalos, A. Papageorgiou et al. 2008 Spironolactone versus eplerenone for the treatment of idiopathic hyperaldosteronism. Expert Opinion Pharmacotherapy. 9:509-515.

46. Kontak AC, Z Wang, D Arbique, B Adams-Huet, RJ Acuchus, SD Nesbitt et al. 2010 Reversible sympathetic overactivity in hypertensive patients with primary aldosteronism Expert Opinion on Pharmacotherapy. 95:4756-4761.

47. Lucatello B, A Benso, I Tabaro, E Capelo, MP Caprino, L Marafetti et al. 2013 European Journal of Endocrinology. 168:525-532.

48. Luther JM. 2014 Effects of aldosterone on insulin sensitivity and secretion. Steroids. 91:54-60.

49. Martins JM, SD Vale, AF Marins. 2014 Mild adrenal steroidogenic defects and ACTH-dependent aldosterone secretion in high blood pressure: preliminary evidence. International Journal of Endocrinology. doi: 10.1155/2014/295724.

50. Marzano L, G Colussi, LA Sechi, C Catena. 2014 Adrenalectomy is comparable with medical treatment for reduction of left ventricular mass in primary aldosteronism: meta-analysis of long-term studies. American Journal of Hypertension. 28(3):312-318.

51. McManus RJ, J Mant, MS Haque et al. Effect of self-monitoring and medication self-titrating on systolic blood pressure in hypertensive patients at high risk of cardiovascular disease: the TASMIN-SR randomized clinical trial. JAMA. 312:799-808.

52. Mehta AN, A Fenves. 2010 Current opinions in renovascular hypertension. Proceedings Baylor University Medical Center. 23:246-249.

53. Melin B, JP Eclache, G Geelen et al. 1980 Plasma AVP, neurophysin, renin activitiy, and aldosterone during submaximal exercise performed until exhaustion in trained and untrained men. European Journal of Applied Physiology and Occupational Physiology. 44:141-151.

54. Milliez P, X Girerd, PF Plouin, J Blacher, ME Safar, JJ Mourad. 2005 Evidence for an increased rate of cardiovascular events in patients with primary aldosteronism. Journal of American College of Cardiology. 45:1243-1248.

55. Mozaffarian D, EJ Benjamin, AS Go, et al. 2015 Heart disease and stroke statistics- 2015 update: a report from the American Heart Association. Circulation. 131 epub.

56. Muldowney JAS, JA Schoenhard, CD Benge. 2009 The clinical pharmacology of eplerenone. Expert Opinion Drug Metabolic Toxicology. 5:425-432.

57. Muth A, O Ragnarsson, G Jahannsson, B Wangberg. 2015 Systematic review of surgery and outcomes in patients with primary aldosteronism. British Journal of Surgery. published ahead of print January 20, 2015.

58. O'Donnell, M, A Mente, S Rangarajan, MJ McQueen, X Wang, L Liu et al. 2015 Urinary sodium and potassium excretion, mortality and cardiovascular events. The New England Journal of Medicine. 371:612-623.

59. Parthasarathy HK, J Menard, WB White, et al. 2011 A double-blind, randomized study comparing the antihypertensive effect of eplerenone and spironolactone in patients with hypertension and evidence of primary aldosteronism. Journal of Hypertension. 29:980-990.

60. Petramala L, L Zinnamosca, A Settevendemmie et al. 2014 Bone and

mineral metabolism in patient with primary aldosteronism. International Journal of Endocrinology. 836529 doi.

61. Pimenta E, RD Gordon, AH Ahmed, D Cowley, R Leano, TH Marwick et al. et al. 2011 Cardiac dimensions are largely determined by dietary salt in patients with primary aldosteronism: results of a case-control study. Journal of Clinical Endocrinology and Metabolism. 96:2813-2820.

62. Pimenta E, RD Gordon, M Stowasser. 2013 Salt, aldosterone and hypertension. Journal of Human Hypertension. 27:1-6.

63. Raman SP, M Lessne, S Kawamoto, Y Chen, R Salvatori, JD Prescott et al. 2015 Diagnostic performance of multidetector computed tomography in distinguishing unilateral from bilateral abnormalities in primary hyperaldosteronism: comparison of multidetector computer tomography with adrenal vein sampling. Journal of Computer Assisted tomography. January, Epub ahead of print.

64. Rankin JW. 2015 Effective diet and exercise interventions to improve body composition in obese individuals. American Journal of Lifestyle Medicine. January/February:48- 62.

65. Rossi GP, G Bernini, C Caliumi, G Desideri, B Fabris, C Ferri et al. 2006 A prospective study of the prevalence of primary aldosteronism in 1,125 hypertensive patients. Journal of the American College of Cardiology. 48:2293-2300.

66. Shey J, MA Cameron, K Sakhaee, OW Moe. 2004 Recurrent calcium nephrolithiasis associated with primary aldosteronism. American Journal of Kidney Diseases. 44:E7-E12.

67. Shibata H, H Itoh. 2012 Mineralcorticoid receptor-associated hypertension and its organ damage: clinical relevance for resistant hypertension. American Journal of Hypertension. 25:514-523.

68. Sonino N, E Tomba, ML Genesia, C Bertello, P Mulatero, F Veglio et al. 2011 Psychological assessment of primary aldosteronism: a controlled study. Journal of Clinical Endocrinology and Metabolism. 96:E878-883.

69. Stowasser M, AH Ahmed. 2014 Quality-of-life aspects of primary aldosteronism. in Primary Aldosteronism: Molecular genetics,

endocrinology, and translational medicine. P. Hellman editor, Springer publisher pp 197- 208.

70. Tomaschitz A, E Ritz, B Pieske et al. 2012 Aldosterone and parathyroid hormone: a precarious couple for cardiovascular disease. Cardiovascular Research. 94:10-19.

71. Tomaszewski M, C White, P Prashanth, N Masca, R Damani, J Hepworth et al. 2014 High rates of non-adherence to antihypertensive treatment revealed by high-performance liquid chromatography-tandem mass spectrometry (HP LC-MS/MS) urine analysis. Heart. 100:855-861.

72. Velasco A, W Vongpatanasin. 2014 The evaluation and treatment of endocrine forms of hypertension. Current Cardiology Reports. 16:528.

73. Weiner D. 2013 Endocrine and hypertensive disorders of potassium regulation: primary aldosteronism. Seminars in Nephrology. 33:265-276.

74. Yoneda T, M Demura, H Takata et al. 2012 Unilateral primary aldosteronism with spontaneous remission after long-term spironolactone therapy. Journal of Clinical Endocrinology and Metabolism. 97:1109-1113.

75. Zannad F, JJV McMurray, H Krum, DJV Veldhuisen, K Swedberg, H Shi et al. 2011 Eplerenone in patients with systolic heart failure and mild symptoms. The New England Journal of Medicine. 364:11- 21.

76. Zennaro C, S Boulkroun, F Fernandes-Rosa. 2015 An update on novel mechanisms of primary aldosteronism. Journal of Endocrinology. 224:R63-R77.

ABOUT THE AUTHOR

Janet Walberg Rankin has been a professor at Virginia Tech for over 30 years. She teaches classes and does research on the effect of diet and physical activity on health and performance in the department of Human Nutrition, Foods, and Exercise. She is a Fellow and a past President of the American College of Sports Medicine. She lives with her husband in Blacksburg, Virginia and visits her adult twin children. She was unusually healthy until age 58 when she suddenly developed high blood pressure. After months of confusion and ineffective treatment, she discovered her problems were related to aldosteronism. This book is the result of her effort to understand this condition and share her knowledge with others. See her website at: https://primaryaldosteronism.wordpress.com/.

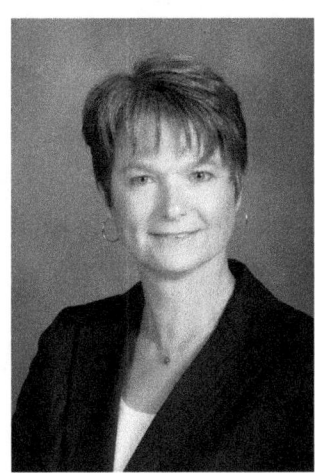